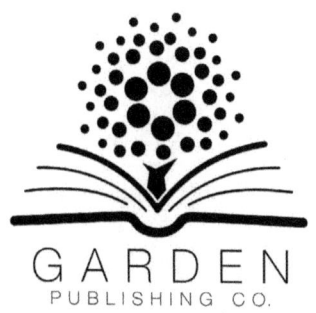

www.gardenpublishingco.com

LIBERATED

KEVIN MCSPADDEN
DESTROYING THE SPIRITUAL CHAINS OF
PORNOGRAPHY AND BONDGAE

Copyright ©2018 by Kevin McSpadden
Published by Garden Publishing Company LLC
For more information, please visit gardenpublishingco.com

All rights reserved. No parts of this publication may be reproduced, stored in a retrieval system, or transmitted in any form or by any means, electronic, mechanical, photocopying, recording, or otherwise, without the prior written permission of the copyright owner.

This book is sold subject to the condition that it shall not, by way of trade or otherwise, be lent, resold, hired out, or otherwise circulated without the publisher's prior consent in any form of binding or cover other than that in which it is published and without a similar condition including this condition being imposed on the subsequent purchaser. Under no circumstances may any part of this book be photocopied for resale.

Scripture taken from the New King James Version of the Bible ©. Used by Permission, all rights reserved.

ISBN 978-0-9966453-4-8
Cover design by Garden Publishing Co./Whitney Whitt
Interior design by Garden Publishing Co.
Illustrated by Whitney Whitt

Printed in the United States of America.

DEDICATION

This book is dedicated to the liberating work of the Holy Spirit and to all those who have committed themselves to pursuing His freedom. It is His fervent desire to put an end to the stronghold of pornography in the beloved bride of Jesus. May we rise to fulfill the Spirit's call to purity.

TABLE OF CONTENTS

Note from the Author	p. 9
Introduction	p. 13
Part One: Do Not Be Deceived	p. 23
Part Two: Blessed to Endure	p. 49
Part Three: Stand Fast	p. 71
Appendix 1: The Gospel: Step One to Freedom	p. 103
Appendix 2: Deliverance Ministry: We Do Not Struggle Against Flesh and Blood	p. 109
To the Wives and Family Members	p. 119

NOTE FROM THE AUTHOR

Dear Reader,

I'm writing this not as someone who pretends to have all the answers about an issue that is both very complex and very devastating, but as one who has walked through all the issues about which I'm writing and who is willing to share what I've learned. It is my hope that this book empowers and encourages you in your own journey with Jesus, and that the revelations I'm sharing from my life will help you walk in greater freedom.

Although this book comes from my experiences specifically with pornography, these revelations about how the spirit of bondage works will be useful for anyone trying to break free from any form of bondage or addiction. In other words, don't put this book down just because you're not necessarily struggling with pornography. If you deal with things like constant anger, any form of addiction (television, food, alcohol, drugs, etc.), or any consistent and familiar form of temptation, you'll find something here to help you.

Furthermore, a common assumption is that only men struggle with pornography. The truth is that many women also deal with this issue. Therefore, even though I am primarily writing this to my brothers in Christ, the truths contained in this book will be very powerful for the sisters as well.

It is also important to understand that I'm writing this with the assumption that you've received Jesus as your Lord and Savior, that you're familiar with deliverance from demonic oppression, and that you've been baptized in the Holy Spirit. If any of those is lacking in your faith walk, I recommend that you start there. The appendices at the back of this book cover the basics of salvation, deliverance ministry, and the baptism of the Holy Spirit for those who want to look into those essential parts of true freedom. They also refer to sources for more information.

The truths I'm sharing in this book will be helpful to you, but ultimate victory always comes by the power of the Holy Spirit. If you're missing that, you never stood a chance in the first place. Also, to tear down a stronghold without removing the ungodly spirit that built that stronghold is an exercise in futility, and it will leave you stuck in the cycles you're trying to escape. I'm just being honest with you, which is what we all need – honesty with ourselves and others.

> **FREEDOM:**
>
> *For our purposes, freedom means the degree to which someone demonstrates Christ-like character. Consider true freedom as being 100% what God intends you to be and 0% anything else. It is both something granted to us upon salvation, since we're freed from our old captivity to sin (see Romans 6), and something we continue to allow Holy Spirit to develop.*

Consider this your fair warning: I'm not going to sugar coat the realities I experienced or the truth of what it takes to get free from bondage. When Jesus taught me these principles and practical steps, He did it in a way that was both painful and loving. He did not do me any disservice by allowing me to hold on to any of the illusions I had previously clung to, nor did He cause me to feel condemned. He allowed me to see the seriousness of what I had done, but He also demonstrated the greatness of His love and mercy to me.

This combination of the love and the seriousness of God is the full picture all believers need to understand if we are going to live truly free from the power of bondage. We have to behold both the goodness and the severity of the Lord

(Romans 11:22 and 2 Corinthians 5:10-11). Then we can approach Him with both the humility and the confident hope that allow Him to truly transform us. I will do my best to represent both of these to you, and it is my prayer that Holy Spirit will grant me grace to do so.

Ultimately, the purpose of this book is encouragement, edification, and exhortation. If you're feeling condemned as you read, please realize that the voice you're hearing is not the voice of Jesus. He never condemns; He does speak the truth in love, even when it is painful to hear. That being said, I encourage you not to give in to shame, guilt, or condemnation, since those things never produce any good fruit. Silence those voices and invite Jesus to speak to you as only He can.

> **WEAPONS OF OUR WARFARE:**
>
> *Silencing the voice of the enemy involves two parts. First, we take authority over those words and through prayer, cast them down. Second, we speak the truth over ourselves. It's not enough to ignore a voice, especially if it keeps on nagging you. Tell it to be silent in Jesus name, then speak what Scripture says about you.*

Finally, please embrace the correction of the Lord as it comes to you. He never disciplines us for destruction, but so that we can be more like Him. He wants us to win. No champion ever experienced victory without training. It hurts, but it's worth it.

For the sake of your marriage, your reputation, your ministry, your call, and your destiny, I encourage you to humble yourself before the Lord. Listen carefully to what He wants you to take from what you're about to read, and most importantly, obey Him fully. May He teach you, guide you, and reveal Himself to you.

In His Grace and Mercy,
Kevin McSpadden

PRAYER:

Father God,

In the name of Jesus, I ask You to teach me through Your Word, Your Holy Spirit, and through this book. Quicken my heart to all You want me to receive as I read. I ask for the Spirit of Truth to guide me into all truth. I ask for the freedom Jesus purchased for me at the cross to manifest fully in my life. Heal me, deliver me, discipline me, and fill me with Your mighty love. I submit myself to You and I receive all that You have planned for me. Thank You for all You will do in my life. In the name of Jesus, Amen.

> **WEAPONS OF OUR WARFARE:**
>
> *Humbling ourselves means we obey what God's written and revealed word say to do. Pride says "I want," while humility says, "yes, Lord."*

John 16:13 -- "However, when He, the Spirit of truth, has come, He will guide you into all truth; for He will not speak on His own authority, but whatever He hears He will speak; and He will tell you things to come."

INTRODUCTION

Twenty years. In some ways, that's a pretty staggering number. The particular twenty-year period I'm referring to saw five presidential elections. It encompassed two separate Middle East wars. It saw the turning of a millennium. In these two decades, I graduated high school and college, became a teacher and coach, and met the woman of my dreams. I came to know Jesus as Savior and Lord. I found an amazing church body that equipped me to thrive in the Kingdom of Jesus. I played drums on two worship cd's. I wrote a book about my personal relationship with God. I became a leader in our congregation. And I was addicted to pornography the entire time.

Twenty years.

They say truth hurts, and I'll admit that coming to terms with the fact that I spent twenty years of my life tangled up in the sticky and seductive web of pornography was a pretty stout slap in the face of my pride. I suppose that's actually a good thing, since pride is one of the reasons I stayed caught so long, but it hurts nevertheless. To look at my life and realize that I was hooked on porn longer than I went to school, college included – the level of disappointment I have felt in myself is hard to describe. It is truly devastating to have to admit such a thing.

But a believer really can't dwell on past sins and failures. It is true that to really get free from bondage, you first have to see it for what it is. Nevertheless, it is also true that the forgiveness and mercy of God are so much greater than our rebellious ways that He can completely redefine our identities and make those things of which we are ashamed as though they never happened. **What a miracle to be able to acknowledge what I've done without being ruled or controlled by it!** How amazing to reflect on something so heinous without condemnation or guilt! How great is the mercy of my God.

It's from the place of one who has desperately needed and overwhelmingly received God's mercy that I write. This is my act of love and service, my labor of gratitude to Jesus. I'm thankful for what He has accomplished in my life and for what He continues to accomplish on a daily basis. That's why I can sit and write what I'm writing: not because I'm good, but because He's truly great.

And this is not an easy thing to put on paper for the world to see. This is my heart, after all. I'm opening it up for you to see, flaws and all. This is the chest where for most of my life I've locked away an intimate, embarrassing secret, and I'm flinging the lid wide open. This is my reputation, and I'm tossing it on the altar because in doing so, I'm praying and believing that Jesus will use my testimony and the understanding He has given me to help break you free in whatever area you need it.

So let me tell you a little bit about the person writing this so you can at least get the basic idea of where I've been. I first discovered the murky realm of pornography as an unsuspecting twelve year old. Up late one night with a friend, we found a channel that aired adult content after ten at night. I'd like to think that, had I known what the horrific consequences would be for years (or decades) to come, I'd have just said "no thanks" and steered clear of that catastrophe. But I didn't know. I just watched with clueless fascination. Like a fish chasing a lure, by the time I figured out what I had gotten ahold of, the hooks were already set, and I was well on my way to the frying pan.

And thus began what would become a raging battle in my life. At the age of seventeen, when I first received Jesus as Lord, I had already been struggling with this addiction for years. That day at the altar, I first encountered the boundless mercy of Jesus as He received me to Himself, and the release I felt as He laid hold of me for His own was like nothing I had ever experienced. In that wave of love, I laid down my old addiction... for a time. But then I went back.

As a college student, I felt like a huge hypocrite. I had a genuine love for the Word of God and for sharing my faith in Jesus, but I continually felt the need to hide what I saw as a glaring flaw in my Christian image. Eventually, I slowly wandered away from church gatherings so that at least I didn't have to pretend I had it all together when the truth was I felt like the only one around struggling with such serious evil.

> **📖 STRONGHOLD:**
>
> *a place where the believer has surrendered authority to the enemy; a pattern of thoughts, behaviors, or words that has power and gains more power the longer a believer allows it to exist. Think of it as a place where demonic spirits can "live," or occupy space in your life.*

After college, as I began my teaching career, I experienced true revival for the first time. God placed me in the midst of believers who were after His heart and actually lived as though He were the most important part of their lives. With these saints as my companions, I rediscovered my first love. I soared. I even came to understand that hiding my addiction would never release me from it. But still I kept my filthy secret.

My life gradually became a predictable cycle. I proceeded from spiritual high, to apathetic lull, to temptation, to willful participation with sin, to depression. In the depression phase, I often went on pornographic binges, trying to compensate for the hatred I felt toward myself. How sick it is to hate what you're doing and still completely give yourself to it! After I spent some time wallowing in sin, God would break through with His reassuring voice. He still loved me. He still wanted me. The cycle would begin its upward trend.

I would pursue Jesus passionately in worship and in His Word. I would vow never to go back to the disgusting secret I kept hidden in the dark. But I did. The cycle repeated.

Upon discovering deliverance ministry, I was elated to learn that I was not the only factor at work in this equation. I learned what strongholds truly were, and that spirits, while they never possessed a believer, could gain authority to operate in our lives. With that new understanding, I felt I had been given a key that had been missing all along. I enthusiastically went through my first deliverance with my friends, the Caldwells, and I experienced a new degree of freedom in the Lord. Not long after, I was baptized in the Holy Spirit, and I truly felt like a new creation.

But you guessed it – I stumbled yet again. This time, I didn't just hide from believers, I ran. I spent a period of about four months in outright rebellion against God. I never set foot inside a church door. I did not abandon my faith in Jesus, but I refused to serve Him or be around His people. You see, I thought I had blown it. I didn't understand at that point in my life that deliverance is not an event, but a lifestyle. Yet even in that dark valley of my life, Jesus pursued me. His love won again.

In 2009, I entered the Garden Supernatural Training Center. I also met my beautiful and amazing wife, Karen, that year. We married in 2010, and by 2011, I had completed the two years of ministry training available through the Garden STC. I was playing drums in the Garden worship team, Rivers Rising, and was serving in a leadership role with the Garden Gathering, which was in its fledgling phase as a church. Around that time, I published my first book, *Average Christians Don't Exist: Encouragement for Believers.* God was empowering me to fulfill my destiny.

And somehow, in the middle of all these wonderful life events, I still managed to deceive myself. Despite my growth in the knowledge and power of the Spirit, I had occasional bouts of temptation toward porn. I even stepped into it two or three times. I was always grieved and guilt-ridden over it. I knew it was a violation of Karen's trust and my marriage vows. I knew to pray for forgiveness, repent to the Lord and to my wife, cast out spirits at work, and receive cleansing. But I still denied that I was entertaining this familiar old addiction. I chalked it up to the notion that all guys struggle in this area and I was bound to stumble now and again.

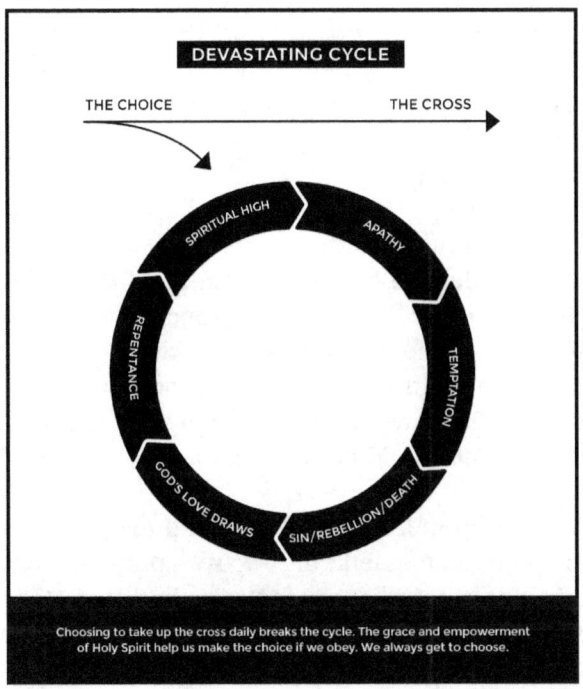

So I did. In May of 2015 I found myself once again in full blown participation with pornography, masturbation, fantasies – the whole stinking stronghold in full operation. And this time, Holy Spirit was not playing games – or rather, He was not allowing me to play games.

In the past, when I "slipped up," as I tritely thought of it, I cruised through the guilt-repent-move on routine. This time, I was led to open up fully to Karen about what was going on in my heart. She was taken completely by surprise, since I had recently informed her that I felt stronger than I ever had in this area. In that previous conversation, I had basically claimed that I had dealt with my pornography habit and that I was not really struggling with it any more. I had allowed pride to blind me to some very obvious weak spots. The reality was that in my mind, through fantasies, scenarios, or simple ungodly recall of the things I had seen, I had never genuinely put the desire for or pleasure from pornography to death.

> **WEAPONS OF OUR WARFARE:**
>
> *God has given us tools and weapons that work to destroy the enemy's power. It is up to use to USE those weapons by the direction of the Holy Spirit.*

And so, under the intense conviction of the Holy Spirit, I admitted all these things to her, expecting a quick release and easy forgiveness. She was gracious. She forgave me. She even reaffirmed her faith in me as a man of God. Nevertheless, I had wounded her deeply, and the weeks and months to come would be some of the most difficult in our marriage.

It didn't stop there. After I met with my pastor, Brandy Helton, and confessed my active participation with pornography, masturbation, fantasies, etc., the Holy Spirit counseled her that I would need to "sit down" from all ministry activities for three months. It was a time to be set apart for Him, to receive healing, and to hear what He would teach me. In addition, as I confessed to Grant and Amber Hill, the worship pastors I served with, I learned I would be sitting down from the worship team during that three month period as well.

To top it all off, Holy Spirit pressed upon Brandy that I needed to write letters to the Garden leadership team and worship team confessing my sin and explaining why I would not be in ministry for the upcoming months. That resonated with me as well. It was not punishment. Rather, it was for the sake of opening up and receiving the forgiveness of my brothers and sisters in Christ. Nevertheless, writing these letters was a humbling task.

So there I was being disciplined, with three months of no ministry activity in front of me. It also happened to be summer vacation, which, for a teacher like me, meant even more time to be with Jesus and allow Him to teach me. I approached that time with as humble and open a heart as I had ever approached anything, and what God did in me during those months was as powerful as it was painful.

In His perfect way, He first set about tearing down the delusions I had entertained about my level of freedom. It came as a series of pointed questions. Did I have authority? *Yes.* Did I have some knowledge and ability in spiritual warfare? *Yes.* Was I growing in the knowledge of God and being raised up in His image? *You bet!* Did I have a tendency to entertain ungodly thoughts that led to temptation? *Oops.* Was there at least some small part of me that wanted to keep the pornography around? *No...maybe...apparently so.* Had I ever been fully honest with myself about what I took from pornography or why it appealed to me? *Uh, nope.* Had I ever fully meant it when I said I wanted to be free? *Dang!* Was I willing to face the truth about why those temptations lingered? (*Stunned silence.*)

The Holy Spirit did not spare His rod as He revealed the evil desires I had harbored in my heart for so many years. I had no choice but to admit that I still took delight in these false lovers of porn and fantasy and physical pleasure. With His light shining on my heart, I could not help but admit that I had always reserved just a tiny measure of my affection for these old, familiar friends of mine. I became disgusted with myself. Only His grace kept me from heaping condemnation upon my head.

From that first step, He proceeded to reveal the true nature of pornography and all that goes with it. When I gave myself to pornography, it wasn't a "slip up," it was a deliberate action brought about because of days, weeks, or possibly months of self-deception that culminated in outright participation. Furthermore, it wasn't an issue that only affected me, as I was fond of telling myself. My participation with defilement had the power to pollute all I came in contact with. And most painful of all to realize, this act of selfishness was not a "minor offense," as some are prone to believe. It was sexual fulfillment outside my marriage. In the eyes of my Redeemer and Judge, it was an act of adultery.

Until that time, I only thought I understood brokenness. Knowing in my heart that I had committed the sin of adultery against my beloved Karen and against my King Jesus destroyed the last shred of dignity I had tried to maintain, along with the illusions I had propped up with my flimsy logic. I was an adulterer. Period.

> **WEAPONS OF OUR WARFARE:**
>
> ***Choice.*** *Our choices determine what power operates in our lives. Choosing to obey God makes us free from sin's power and helps us grow in His. Submitting to sin increases its power over us. The constant choice to obey God is a mighty weapon in our arsenal.*

I had no claim upon the mercy of God except what He in His goodness was willing to pour upon me. I had no claim upon Karen's love, trust, or affection except what the Holy Spirit worked in her heart to give me. I deserved none of it; I was in the position of complete dependence.

Praise God for grace.

From the position of dependence and humility, God was able to teach me. He met me in the brokenness, pouring out new and fresh understanding. He raised me up from the depths of condemnation and reaffirmed my identity as His son, His chosen vessel. He showed me the weapons of my warfare that I had neglected. He even taught me how to cover and defend what could be weak places. And He taught me the real value of dependence on Him. Like many Christians, men especially, I had resisted becoming vulnerable before the Lord because it made me feel weak. The reality was quite the opposite: maintaining a dependence upon the

Spirit kept me humble, and it helped keep my eyes open. Dependence on and submission to Him actually made me stronger. When my time of discipline was finished, He set me back in my place as a fully healed, newly transformed man.

And then, after giving me some time to truly walk in the new revelation He had given me, He released me to share what He had done in my life with others. **I believe life-changing transformation is available to every person who will lay hold of it**. Ultimately, our God is the God of victory, and His children are blessed to walk with Him in that victory in every area of our lives.

Do you believe it?

Much of what you are about to read comes directly from what I received from the Lord during my time of discipline. Some of it, He gave me later, since He always continues to refine our understanding and reveal to us the deeper truths. That's the Holy Spirit's job after all, and He's really good at it. I know He will continue to teach me in the days to come.

So here we go. I can honestly say that I cannot think of anyone less qualified to write this book than I am. And yet, I know in my heart that I was called to do it. It is the Lord who has qualified us to carry His message, and sometimes, the only qualification we have is our "yes" in response to His command.

This is my "yes."

LIBERATED

PART ONE: DO NOT BE DECEIVED

It's a Command

The first chapter of James describes the process by which temptation leads to sin and finally death. Take a moment to read James 1:12-18. I'll be re-visiting this passage many times as we move forward, but for now, after you've read the whole passage, focus in on verse sixteen.

After James (by inspiration of the Holy Spirit) describes how temptation leads to sin and death, he gives the command: "Do not be deceived." Whenever you see a command in Scripture, understand that God does not command us to do things unless He knows we can do it. **More accurately, He only commands us to do what He intends to provide us the power to accomplish.** He's a perfect Father and Lord, so He does not command us in order to frustrate us or cause us to fail. He commands us so that we can put His glory on display as we accomplish what would be impossible without Him.

Keeping that in mind, the command, "Do not be deceived," indicates that there is both an option and an empowerment involved. The option is in our choice. Will we choose to listen to and obey the truth, or will we give in to the lie? Assuming that our answer is that we prefer the truth, the other side of the equation is the grace God gives us to carry out what He has commanded. In other words, God has empowered us to see, recognize, and live in the truth. If we are not living in truth, it is very likely due to our own choices. It is true that unbelievers have their minds blinded from truth. However, a Christian who has received the Holy Spirit of Truth and who has the mind of Christ generally only becomes deceived when we fail to listen to and/or obey what God has spoken, either through His revealed or written Word.

This is especially clear because the Bible provides vivid and plain descriptions of how the process of deception works. The passage we read from James chapter one takes away all the mystery: first we entertain evil desire, then we're enticed, then we sin, and sin leads us to death. It's not complicated. Reading it on this page, you're probably wondering how we ever give in to this stuff in the first place. But it happens, and it happens primarily as a result of deception.

EVIL DESIRE	GOOD DESIRE
Based on self-pleasure; selfishness	Based on pleasing the Lord; service
Comes from flesh or attention to ungodly things	Comes from abiding in Him
Produces bad fruit, ultimately death	Produces good fruit for all
Opposes God's Word and calling	Lines up with God's Word and His calling on my life
Keeps my attention toward sin	Moves my attention toward the Lord

It usually starts when we deceive ourselves in some way. Whether it is with anger or lust or abuse or addiction or whatever it may be, deception cloaks our eyes in every step as temptation leads us toward destruction. I'll illustrate with some of my experiences during my struggle with pornography.

In the "before" phase, where temptation is just beginning, the deception stops us from admitting that what we're craving at that moment is wrong. We fail to recognize that the desire we're experiencing is in fact an evil desire. For someone who has walked with the Lord any time at all, evil desires should be fairly easy to recognize, but deception attempts to cloud the waters and blur the lines we know better than to cross. If I asked any husband, "Do you think it's right to cheat on your wife, count her love as worthless, and prefer another woman over her?" I know what the answer would be. It's easy right? Well that's where deception whispers in our ears and convinces us otherwise.

See if any of these statements sound familiar: *What you're wanting is justified. Your wife was rude to you. She hasn't taken care of your needs. It's only natural. You need release and it's okay to take care of yourself. You would never really touch another woman, and this isn't the same thing. You want to do this. Why shouldn't you do this? You'll feel better if you do this.*

I could go on listing lies, but I won't. The point is that all of these sentiments blur and hide what should be plainly obvious: What you're thinking about or being tempted by is sin, which is bad. Your heart is not for it. You know God hates it. It is evil. Period.

And yet, we still get to choose. If we are "enticed," as James put it, that means we have

> **RENOUNCE:**
>
> *According to Dictionary.com, to renounce something means:*
> 1. *to give up or put aside voluntarily.*
> 2. *to give up by formal declaration.*
> 3. *to repudiate; disown.*
>
> *In other words, you renounce something when you willfully decide to put it away and give up ownership or participation with it.*

given our attention to something we knew was evil. It is our choice. We're not overcome by temptation; we willingly submit to it. How do I know that? Jesus set us free from the power of sin (Romans 6:2). If we're sinning, it's not because we have to. If we're tempted, it usually means we are giving something our attention that has no business in our thoughts or sight. After all, you can't be enticed by something that you don't focus on.

If you're sitting outside a bakery with a blindfold on and your nose plugged up, you probably won't feel the need to run in and eat cookies. You're oblivious to the fact that they're even being baked. But yank that blindfold off and pull that plug. You see the sign and notice the rows of delicious-looking goodies. You take in that aroma. Now you have to make effort NOT to go eat cookies.

It's a simple illustration of a powerful truth: **once something has your attention, it has the ability to stir your desire. Once you truly desire something, it's really just a question of time and opportunity before you pursue it.**

So with temptation, we become deceived when we fail to acknowledge and renounce an evil desire. The power of desire only gets stronger when it has our attention. Then it stops feeling like an itch and starts feeling more like a hook. The battle is on!

> **◣ WEAPONS OF OUR WARFARE:**
>
> *Secrecy is never the right choice when it comes to temptation or sin. Secrecy tends to lead to isolation. Divide and conquer is one of the oldest - and most effective - plays in the enemy's book.*

Then, deception continues as we ponder committing the actual sinful act. In this phase, deception can make it seem like we're justifying what we're doing, even though it's pretty obvious that it's wrong: *This will be the last time. Never again. This is just a little wrong. It's not like I'm killing someone. Everyone does this. I'll just ask for forgiveness and it'll be okay.*

Again, someone who is not blinded by evil desire can see right through these flimsy facades. All of those thoughts (or similar ones) amount to saying, "I'll slap God directly in the face, then ask for forgiveness." What about that is okay?

Even after the act, deception continues to speak: *I'm only hurting myself. Nobody needs to know. This was not a big deal. I should keep this to myself. I need to hide this so nobody finds out. I can't tell anyone.*

Or, ironically, after we sin, the deceiver will often use the exact opposite of his own temptation to try to condemn us: *I'm worthless. Nobody sins as much or does things as bad as I do. I'm the worst Christian/spouse/parent/human being ever. I'm the only one who struggles with this.*

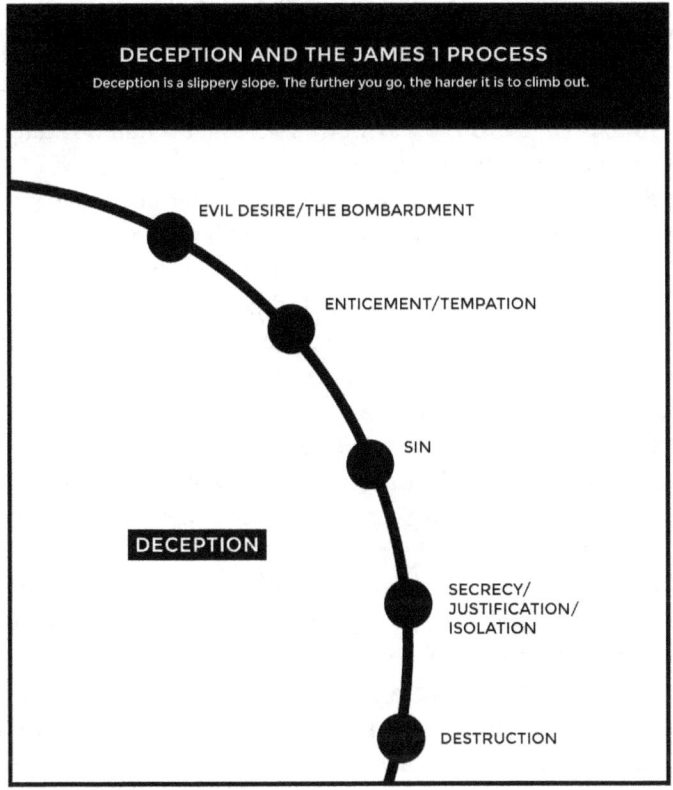

At every phase, the purpose of deception is to trick, scare, or threaten the one struggling so that they feel they must keep their sin to themselves. As I'll share later, opening up about our struggles is one of the best ways to destroy the power they have. But deception urges us to hide under a cloak of secrecy, which only adds to the torment of it. It's disgusting, but that's how the enemy works.

Unfortunately though, the devil is rarely the only one who has tricked us. Most of the time, we have also deceived ourselves. It starts with the desire, which we choose to accept rather than renounce and rebuke. Then we give it our attention and are enticed. We are worn down until we choose to participate. Finally, active participation with sin hardens our hearts toward God, our friends and family, and ultimately ourselves, and leads us down the path of destruction.

That's the bad news. The good news is we always have a choice. The even better news is that God has not left us defenseless against this temptation.

Romans 6:12-14 says, "Therefore do not let sin reign in your mortal body, that you should obey it in its lusts. And do not present your members as instruments of unrighteousness to sin, but present yourselves to God as being alive from the dead, and your members as instruments of righteousness to God. For sin shall not have dominion over you, for you are not under law but under grace."

Romans 6:16 says, "Do you not know that to whom you present yourselves slaves to obey, you are that one's slaves whom you obey, whether of sin leading to death, or of obedience leading to righteousness?"

James 1:21 says, "Therefore lay aside all filthiness and overflow of wickedness, and receive with meekness the implanted word, which is able to save your souls."

Each of these passages demonstrates clearly that we have a choice in the matter. Satan has no power to *force* us to do anything. He can threaten, lie, cheat, steal, shoot arrows, or try any number of tactics, but our actions still lie entirely within our own will. We can focus on the evil and allow it to consume us, or we can lay it aside, present ourselves to God, and live as instruments of righteousness. Furthermore, we know that God has given us grace to do those very things.

The key to overcoming deception is a focus on the Father and a willingness to obey Him rather than ourselves (or our desires). James 1:17 instructs us, "Every good gift and every perfect gift is from above, and comes down from the Father of lights, with whom there is no variation or shadow of turning."

Put another way, this verse could say, "If it's good, it is from God. Since He is constant, you'll know whether or not He approves of it. If He doesn't approve of it, kill your desire for it, because it's no good." That's my paraphrase, obviously, but it's still a good test: is what I'm desiring of the Lord? If not, then I must choose not to give it my attention. The very second I entertain desires that are not of the Lord, I have opened myself to deception. We know very well where that leads.

Proverbs 7 – The Path of Destruction

Proverbs 7 is a lengthy illustration of where temptation ultimately leads. Consider this chapter both a parable and a warning. The Lord has long known that one of the highlighted maneuvers in the devil's book of tactics is to lure people away with sexual enticement. For a point of reference, Proverbs was written almost 3,000 years ago, and the enemy is still using the same tactic with quite a bit of success, unfortunately. That does not speak well of many of us believers. Nevertheless, let's journey briefly through this chapter for a picture of the path pornography and lust can set a person on.

> **WEAPONS OF OUR WARFARE:**
>
> **Obedience.** *Ever notice how often obedience or the lack thereof makes all the difference? That's why Jesus gave us the model: I speak what I hear my Father speaking; I do what I see Him doing. If it worked for Jesus...*

First, the chapter begins with an exhortation to keep the commands of the father. Spiritually speaking, it is not hard to see that we are the ones spoken to as "my son," while the father represents God and/or the Holy Spirit. The first five verses could be summarized as an encouragement from a father to his children, saying, "Obey me *with your heart* and you won't fall into the trap of the immoral woman." That seems simple enough. However, the rest of the chapter uses one unfortunate young man as an illustration of why we must obey from the heart the instruction we have received.

Verse seven describes the father's vision of a "young man devoid of understanding." In other words, he's a foolish young person who either has not been taught properly, or who has ignored the teachings of God. This young man sets himself up for destruction when he takes the street near an immoral woman's corner and then heads down the path to her house during the evening hours approaching darkness (Proverbs 7:8). Interpreted for our purposes, this man was walking where a believer knows better than to walk. He was providing an opportunity for the flesh (Romans 13:14) by putting himself in a place where temptation was known to live. The context of this passage makes clear that others knew this woman to be immoral, yet he took the roads that led him near her house first, then took the path that led right up to it. The dark evening represents trying to hide what one is doing, yet it is obvious the father still sees him. In the end, the man described in the passage did something he knew he had no business doing.

> **WEAPONS OF OUR WARFARE:**
>
> *Know your weaknesses and act accordingly. If you're aware of how you might be tempted, you have the power to remove that option from the table. Enough said.*

The parallels between this young man and believers struggling with bondage are striking. He walked on a street where an immoral woman lived. We put ourselves in the position to be tempted when we give things our attention that we know could lead to sin. He took the road to the immoral woman's house. We entertain thoughts, memories, and fantasies we know will stir our desire even more. He tried to go in the dark evening. We try to hide our true intentions from others and ourselves, but the Father is not blinded to what we're doing.

From verse ten through twenty, the immoral woman begins her seduction of the simple young man. Her clothes, her scent, and her words are all designed to entice him toward sin. Sights, scents, sounds, and sensations are all invoked in her seduction. Her harlot's attire is designed to catch the eye. Her description of perfumes lure him in with pleasant smells. Her sultry voice tempts him to lower his defenses. Her descriptions of soft tapestry and a bed whose rightful owner is away appeal to the young man's fleshly lust. By the time she finishes, the young man is caught by hooks he doesn't even know are there.

This part demonstrates the importance of recognizing and shutting down whatever form of temptation comes at us. The eyes, ears, nose, and bodily sensations all have the ability to snag our attention if we are unaware or unwilling to admit what is happening. It is hard to say when a sound, for example, may remind us of something we've heard that can spark enticement. However, once we recognize a desire in operation, we have to cut it off before it takes us anywhere. In the Proverbs 7 passage, the young man would have done well to run away like his life depended on it, but instead, he remained and talked to the temptress, sealing his fate. Likewise, we do well to flee from lusts (2 Timothy 2:22), but to remain focused on temptation is folly.

The next part of Proverbs 7 shows the real intention of the spirits of whoredom and bondage, represented in this passage by the immoral woman. She seduces him and he yields, meaning she doesn't overpower him and take him by force. He chooses to come in with her. His surrender of his attention to her vivid descriptions make him like an ox led to slaughter. This familiar image of an ignorant ox led to its death suggests the devouring appetite of our enemy, who would like nothing more than to slaughter the saints of God. Furthermore, the young man becomes like a fool bound for the stocks, speaking of the humiliation the devil intends to pour out upon those he seduces in this way. The passage also compares the man to a bird heading straight for a snare intended to catch him. He has made himself an easy target.

The chapter finishes with the exhortation to stay focused on the father's words and instruction. Two particular principles stick out: 1. The command not to "let your heart turn aside to her ways" points again to the power desire can have to change our course if we choose to allow it, and 2. The encouragement not to "stray into her paths" suggests that we must choose to keep ourselves away from the places we know temptation dwells.

To illustrate practically, it is extremely unwise for those who have struggled with alcohol addiction to hang out in bars. Is it possible for a former alcoholic to hang out with a friend who is having a drink and remain un-tempted? Absolutely. But I would recommend a serious heart check before doing such a thing simply because that person would be putting himself in immediate proximity with a substance that has severely afflicted his life. If he has victory and the old temptations have no hold, then he is free to do what the Lord allows him to do. Otherwise, he has taken a path he knows leads to destruction.

Put another way, if I know of a place where poisonous snakes live, I would be unwise to sit casually near that den and read a book. The better choice would be to simply go read somewhere else, or to destroy the den before I spent any time near there. Otherwise, I'm putting myself in a position where I'm likely to get bitten. In each scenario, wise behavior and staying away from a known threat help preserve the believer from destruction.

Returning to Proverbs 7, the point of this chapter, at least for our purposes in this book, is that believers have no business putting ourselves in the position to be tempted. The story illustrates that the foolish one took an unwise path, gave his attention and desire to a known harlot, chose to enter her house, and ended up slaughtered. That's the warning from the wise father to those who have ears to hear: "Her house is the way to hell, descending to the chambers of death" (Proverbs 7:27). It can't be made any clearer than that. So why would any believer go near such a place?

Unfortunately, however, many of us do. The story would be a powerful enough warning if the young fool were the only one who had ever done it, but the father tells us, "she has cast down *many wounded,* And all who were slain by her were *strong men*" (Proverbs 7:26, emphasis added). Did you get that, Christians? She has cast down thousands, if not millions, of us with mortal wounds. And all of the ones she took down were strong.

How many heads of former mighty men of God does the enemy have mounted on his wall because of sexual sin? How many ministry tombstones are in the immoral woman's backyard? How many more of our brothers and sisters will she murder before the body of Christ comes together as a whole to execute her in our midst? God only knows.

Nevertheless, this chapter makes it painfully clear how the Lord views this type of sin. It is the way to death and hell. It is the path of destruction. We are to stay away from it at all costs. We must not be deceived.

Call It What It Is

It is pretty common for people to deceive themselves by looking at sinful action in ways that seem less horrific than it really is. **In our efforts to justify ourselves in our hearts, we tend to sugar coat, reduce, or downplay what we've done.** As I mentioned before, that's just a form of deception. So now let's look at the sin of pornography as it really is. Let's strip off the veneer and gaze at it in its ugliness.

Note: Remember, even if pornography is not a struggle for you, a lot of this still applies to whatever area of bondage you deal with. Also, the point of this is not to be harsh, but to be truthful. It's just that in this particular area, the truth is very ugly.

For starters, pornography and masturbation are both sexual acts. You can twist it any way you want, but it doesn't change the truth. "But I'm not participating in the sex when I watch porn." We'll get to this in a moment, but Jesus did not distinguish between active participation and simply looking when He said lust was the same thing as adultery. Secondly, ask yourself whether or not your spouse would be happy to discover you watching other people have sex.

If you're single, ask the same question with Jesus in place of your spouse. Thirdly, in your mind, you're being sexually gratified by what you're watching. If you think you're not, then why do you watch? If you say it's just a picture, why does it have such power to arouse your desire? I could go on, but you get the point. You may not be present in the room where the act is taking place, but you're participating. And as for masturbation, the very definition of that word is sexual self-gratification. In other words, it is sex with yourself, which the Bible never authorizes.

I myself had to come to grips with all of these truths the last time I stepped into the sin of pornography and masturbation. I did not understand why my wife felt so betrayed, and frankly, I couldn't see why it was such a big deal to her. In my mind, these were sins that affected me, but shouldn't really hurt her. She continually tried to explain why my participation with pornography and masturbation had wounded her so deeply, but she was having great difficulty breaking through my self-deception. Finally, in her exasperation with me, she shouted, "Kevin, it is sex and I'm not there!"

At last, the truth became clear.

Holy Spirit confirmed that her feelings are in line with what the Lord sees. First Corinthians 7:4 teaches that spouses have authority over the other's body. **In other words, my wife has the final say over my sexual fulfillment.** When I married her, I surrendered that over to her, and she has authority over it. In her eyes, and in the eyes of Jesus, any sexual act I commit in the absence of my wife, whether I physically touch another woman or not, is a violation of His express order in marriage. Furthermore, 1 Corinthians 6:13 teaches that the body is for the Lord, and the Lord is for the body. He has the primary authority over all that I do with my body, and obviously, I violated both my wife's authority and the direct order of Jesus every time I looked at porn or masturbated.

Even if you're single, there's no way to argue that porn and masturbation (or fantasies, for that matter) are a part of God's plan for sexuality. Jesus Himself made it clear just how seriously God views this topic in Matthew 5:27-28: "You have heard that it was said to those of old, 'You shall not commit adultery.' But I say to you that whoever looks at a woman to lust for her has already committed adultery with her in his heart." According to Jesus's standard, even to look at a woman to lust for her is the same as adultery. Those are His words, not mine, and He did not restrict this standard to married people.

Other places in the Bible discuss the Father's view of sexual immorality, which would include porn, fantasies, masturbation, lust, premarital sex, and adultery. First Corinthians 6:18 says, "Flee sexual immorality. Every sin that a man does is outside the body, but he who commits sexual immorality sins against his own body." This makes it clear that these kinds of sins are committed not only against God Himself, but against our very bodies.

First Corinthians 10:6-11 adds, "Now these things became our examples, to the intent that we should not lust after evil things as they also lusted. And do not become idolaters as were some of them. As it is written, 'The people sat down to eat and drink, and rose up to play.' Nor let us commit sexual immorality, as some of them did, and in one day twenty-three thousand fell; nor let us tempt Christ, as some of them also tempted, and were destroyed by serpents; nor complain, as some of them also complained, and were destroyed by the destroyer. Now all these things happened to them as examples, and they were written for our admonition, upon whom the ends of the ages have come."

So you see, participating with these kinds of sins equates to a very serious issue in the eyes of the Father. Thus far, it has become clear from Scripture that pornography and the other acts that accompany it are identifiable as sexual acts outside marriage, violation of the wife's authority, violation of Jesus's authority, adultery, sexual immorality, and just plain evil.

There are still a few more Scriptural principles I want to highlight. Ephesians 2:1-3 discusses how the lusts of the flesh are a sign of the sons of disobedience. Disobedience may not sound serious, but go back and read the passage above from 1 Corinthians 10. I realize that since the sacrifice of Christ, His grace intervenes for us, but do you still think disobedience is a small offense, considering how God reacted to it in that passage?

If you need further proof of the seriousness of willful disobedience, consider 1 Samuel 15:22-23: "So Samuel said: 'Has the Lord as great delight in burnt offerings and sacrifices, As in obeying the voice of the Lord? Behold, to obey is better than sacrifice, And to heed than the fat of rams. For rebellion is as the sin of witchcraft, And stubbornness is as iniquity and idolatry. Because you have rejected the word of the Lord, He also has rejected you from being king.'" Saul's disobedience cost him his throne. Furthermore, in this same passage the Lord equates rebellion, which is willful disobedience, with witchcraft. God fervently desires His people to wake up and understand the seriousness of constantly disobeying Him. The sons of disobedience will incur the wrath of God, and we want no part of that.

The final reality I want to share is this: to willfully and actively sin is an open insult against Jesus, His precious blood, and the Holy Spirit. Hebrews 10:26-31 tells us, "For if we sin willfully after we have received the knowledge of the truth, there no longer remains a sacrifice for sins, but a certain fearful expectation of judgment, and fiery indignation which will devour the adversaries. Anyone who has rejected Moses' law dies without mercy on the testimony of two or three witnesses. Of how much worse punishment, do you suppose, will he be thought worthy who has trampled the Son of God underfoot, counted the blood of the covenant by which he was sanctified a common thing, and insulted the Spirit of grace? For we know Him who said, 'Vengeance is Mine, I will repay,' says the Lord. And again, 'The Lord will judge His people.' It is a fearful thing to fall into the hands of the living God."

Let me reiterate that my purpose in bringing these truths up is not to condemn, but to dispel illusions and bring clarity. It is not a minor offense to trample the Son of God underfoot, or to consider the blood that set us free worthless, or to insult the Spirit who has empowered us to walk in freedom. **And just to remove any lingering lie about the crucial nature of what we're discussing, let me remind you that it is not your standard by which these sins will be judged, but the standard of Jesus Himself** (Romans 2:16).

Taking all of these principles together, we must call our sin what it is, and as you can see by now, it is horrible, to say the least. Thank God for His immeasurable mercy. I have come to love the mercy of God precisely because I am in need of so much of it!

It is essential, having read these things, that you realize that you are not lost, as long as you hold to your faith in Jesus and what He has done for you. You are not beyond the reach of God's love or mercy. You can and will be forgiven. But you must acknowledge the fullness of what you have done and what you have participated with. Confess to the Lord and He will forgive you and pour His love upon you beyond measure. The parable in Luke 7:41-47 teaches that whoever has been forgiven much, loves much.

My friends, we have been forgiven much. So let us love the Lord enough that we seek not only His forgiveness, but His grace to repent.

Fornication and Murder: Companions in the Lists of Infamy

I'm sure the last part was difficult to read and receive. I know it rocked me as the Lord revealed it to me. Yet, to understand and acknowledge what we have actually done is a major step towards repentance and freedom.

However, I want to take this even a step further. This is one of the things that shocked me the most as the Lord spoke to me during my season of discipline after I last stepped into the sin of pornography. I offer it to you to consider and seek out with Him.

What the Lord showed me is that there is a connection between murder and fornication. As I discussed previously, fornication is sexual immorality, or any of those acts that are not a part of God's plan for sexuality. It was eye-opening to me how many times in Scripture that murder and sexual immorality appear next to each other. Here are some examples.

In Matthew 15:16-20, Jesus corrects the disciples' perception about defilement, stating that it is not what people eat or drink that defiles them. In verses nineteen and twenty, He teaches, "For out of the heart proceed evil thoughts, murders, adulteries, fornications, thefts, false witness, blasphemies. These are the things which defile a man, but to eat with unwashed hands does not defile a man." Notice that adulteries and fornications immediately follow murder on this list of things that defile someone. Also notice that evil thoughts are included on this list. That would include fantasies.

This happens again in Revelation 21:8: "But the cowardly, unbelieving, abominable, murderers, sexually immoral, sorcerers, idolaters, and all liars shall have their part in the lake which burns with fire and brimstone, which is the second death." Once more, we see murderers and the sexually immoral side by side, and this time, Jesus Himself says that such people will have their part in the lake of fire.

Even in the Sermon on the Mount in Matthew 5, Jesus teaches about murder and then follows with teaching on adultery. I'm not saying that these sins are being equated in the Scriptures I've mentioned. I am pointing out that they appear side by side in lists of extremely serious sins, which demonstrates their equal importance. I think it's safe to say that none of us wants to be considered a murderer. But what the Lord emphasized to me is that according to His standard, sexual sin is not necessarily less of a sin than murder. Consider that for yourself.

To further emphasize this point, Ephesians 5:3-6 teaches, "But fornication and all uncleanness or covetousness, let it not even be named among you, as is fitting for saints; neither filthiness, nor foolish talking, nor coarse jesting, which are not fitting, but rather giving of thanks. For this you know, that no fornicator, unclean person, nor covetous man, who is an idolater, has any inheritance in the Kingdom of Christ and God. Let no one deceive you with empty words, for because of these things the wrath of God comes upon the sons of disobedience."

So you see, **fornicators have no inheritance in the Kingdom.** That is a sobering thought.

Now, am I saying that committing these sins will automatically send someone to hell? No. However, I am warning you that these sins are serious and not to be taken lightly. We know that continued participation with sin causes deception and hardens the heart so that eventually the sinner is in danger of rejecting Jesus. That is what will send someone to hell. Therefore, it is crucial that we understand what we're dealing with and repent before it gets to that point. Moreover, we must remember that Satan's ultimate purpose for tempting us toward these sins is to destroy us. Therefore, it is wise to eliminate these influences from our lives so that they have no chance whatsoever to accomplish that goal.

Jesus gave us an important key when He showed us that these sins actually proceed from our *hearts*. The heart is where our relationship with Him really takes place. It is His rightful throne and His home within us.

I do not want Jesus to share His home with murder. In the same way, I want His home to be free from the defilement of sexual immorality in all its forms. And again, that process starts by removing deception and seeing it for what it is.

It Has Never Been ONLY About You

One of the biggest lies that keeps people from repentance and freedom from pornography (or other forms of bondage) is the deception that our sins are only affecting us. "Well if it were hurting someone else," we tell ourselves, "I wouldn't do it. But it's not such a big deal when it's only affecting me."

At face value, that almost sounds noble, as if we were truly looking out for other people by only hurting ourselves. By the time you reach the end of this section, my hope is that you'll see how foolish that way of thinking really is.

After I had come forth and admitted my participation with pornography this last time, I sent a letter to the Garden leadership confessing and asking forgiveness. I received back a great deal of encouragement, prophecy, and edification. Nobody condemned me, and everybody expressed their love. But there was one response in particular that struck my heart so hard I don't think I'll ever forget it.

> **WEAPONS OF OUR WARFARE:**
>
> *Allowing the Holy Spirit to reveal our rightful place in the body of Christ and to show us how God sees us accomplishes two things: 1. It destroys the notion that we're not important to Him. 2. It forces us to humble ourselves as we depend on Him to transform us into the ones He created us to be.*

The e-mail came from a dear sister in the Lord who I've always known to perceive and prophesy with laser accuracy. In her e-mail, she described how she was praying for Karen and me. She reaffirmed her love for us, which we both needed and appreciated. Then came the stunner: the Holy Spirit showed this friend of ours that through my sin, Satan had hit two birds with one stone.

I wish I could tell you I received this message with grace. Instead, I became angry. How dare she write such a disparaging note to me, especially in the midst of my pain and humiliation? What did she know about what my wife and I were going through? I read and re-read the e-mail probably a dozen times. Eventually I just shut off the computer and walked away. But the message would not leave me alone. It kept replaying in my mind until I finally had to acknowledge it and let the Holy Spirit talk to me about it. Lo and behold, our friend was right!

As the days passed, the Spirit opened my eyes to the devastation I had wreaked on Karen. As my wife, she suffered the embarrassment of having her husband admit to participation with pornography, even though she had no part in it whatsoever. She had to come to terms with my rejection of her in favor of internet images. She had to forgive me for preferring a false lover over her intimacy. She lost me as a companion on the worship team during my period of discipline. I had betrayed her trust. I had gone elsewhere for satisfaction. I had wounded her severely, and none of it was her fault!

So yeah, beyond a shadow of a doubt, my sin enabled Satan to hit two birds with one stone. And my situation is not unique. Any sin that we participate in will directly affect our spouses. Ephesians 5:28-31, which is a teaching about Jesus and His church, is also a teaching that the husband and wife are one flesh. Whatever stains one affects the other. It is designed that way. God's intention in marriage was to demonstrate His relationship with us, to offer us intimacy that reflects His love, and to grant us a companion that would encourage, support, and spur us on (and many more amazing benefits than this). However, when we willfully sin, Satan has the opportunity to attack both of us at once.

I had to admit that while my heart's desire would never be to harm my wife in any way, I had done precisely that. And it didn't stop there. One of the most devastating discoveries I made was how my sin affected another of our close friends on our worship team. This woman of God and I have been on the worship team together for years. We've grown up together in the Lord and co-labored in the Kingdom. She and her husband are like family to Karen and me. One day, as I was talking to this friend's husband, he told me that when she found out about my sin, it broke her heart to the point of weeping.

Hearing that only added to the conviction I already felt. I know that my friend's tears were not shed in disappointment or anger, let alone in condemnation of me, but rather out of her genuine love for me. It devastated her see a beloved brother ensnared in this sin. It broke my heart to know that a sister I consider to be pure and genuine was brought to tears on account of her love for me.

On top of that, I put my worship team in a bit of a bind. While we have enough musicians to alternate in and out so that none of us are worn out, we do not yet have so many members that we are not affected when anyone is gone. During my time of discipline and refreshing, the Lord sat me down from being on the worship team. That judgment was absolutely right. God will always protect the purity of His worship, and He had to protect the church body from anything that could come through me to them.

However, it also meant that the other drummers didn't get to rest. It meant that one musician who is usually not a drummer had to leave his normal instrument to stand in for me when the others were gone. Nobody complained, and nobody said a word to me about it. But I saw with my eyes the consequences of my sin. The ministries in which I serve were affected as well, having to make do with one less set of hands to carry out the work.

And none of it was their fault.

I know that not everyone's circumstances are the same as mine, but I use my life as an example to illustrate that the sin with which we participate never affects only us. Jesus calls us His body and says that we are members of one another (Romans 12:4-5). If one part suffers, all of the body suffers because we're connected. There are no parts that can suffer without affecting the others. True, the body still functions by the grace of God, but Jesus is building us up to be like Him. Think of it like this: if you bruise a toe, you don't die, but you sure do feel it. It's harder to walk. It's harder to focus. And that's not even that serious of an injury.

I hope by now you realize the notion that participating with sin only hurts you is completely false. It affects your marriage, your spouse, your ministry, your friendships, and your reputation. Jesus taught that our enemy's job description is to steal, kill, and destroy (John 10:10). How much better for his purposes if he can convince us that he's only after us personally, and not also after all those other wonderful parts of our lives?

I would liken this kind of deception to an assassin. Not that I'm an expert in these matters by any means, but I've never heard of an assassin who was seven feet tall and ran screaming at his victims with a battle axe. Why? Because any person in their right mind would run from such a man or shoot him on sight.

An assassin thrives on *not* being noticed. He is sneaky, deceptive, and uses any means necessary to kill his targets. I would imagine that an assassin considers himself successful if the victim never knows he's there.

> **WEAPONS OF OUR WARFARE:**
>
> *Confessing sin, repenting (committing to yourself and to Jesus that you fully intend to turn away from sin and toward His purposes and plans), and receiving the discipline of the Lord are powerful weapons in your arsenal. While many do not think of these vital acts as warfare, each of them plays a role in restoring your right relationship, both with God and man. Furthermore, they each help you solidify your true identity in Him, which increases your power to overcome the temptation to sin in the future.*

That's how I see this deception working. "There's nothing here," it says. "Go on with what you're doing. Even if someone gets hurt, it's really only you." But once it's in, it goes after everyone and everything you ever cared about. **You wouldn't invite a known killer into your house. So why invite an assassin to cling to your life, looking for chances to kill, steal, and destroy?**

Do you see the selfishness of justifying sin by claiming you're the only one it hurts? To willfully sin is like placing all of these wonderful gifts (including yourself) at the mercy of an assassin simply to engage in a momentary and passing pleasure.

Furthermore, in addition to all these truths, you need to believe that YOU matter! You yourself are important to God. You have a calling. You have a destiny. You have gifts, talents, and dreams that are yours by the will of the Father Himself. No matter how you may feel about yourself after participating with sin, it is NOT okay for you to suffer. Jesus taught that not a sparrow falls from the sky without God's notice, and that we are so much more important than those birds. His eye is on you, and the last thing He wants is for you to suffer. Jesus took our grief, bore our sorrow, paid the price for our sin, took our punishment, and gave us peace because He places that kind of value on *every one of us*.

To agree with the notion that says, "I'm the only one getting hurt, so it's okay," is to disregard the importance placed on your life by God Himself. I'm not preaching pride or arrogance here. In fact, it is arrogant and prideful to believe you know better than God when it comes to deciding how much you're worth. **Humility is to agree with Him regarding your worth and to honor the value He has placed on your life.**

God designed you to carry His love and reflect His glory, and He has not rested for a single second from working in your life. You mean something to Him. Your whole life is a treasure in God's eyes. So please throw away the mindset that would ever justify sinning because "it's only hurting me." You wouldn't throw dirt on a case of fine jewels just because they belonged to you. Neither should you heap filth on yourself. That filth will soil every part of your precious life, whether you mean it to or not. When it comes to your choice about whether or not to engage in willful sin, remember that it has never been about *only* you. Even if it were, it still wouldn't be okay.

My friend, you would do well to value your life, along with all it entails, the same way God does. Ask the Holy Spirit to teach you about your value, and you will never again feel justified in hurting yourself through willful sin.

Confession is Vital; Repentance is a Gift; Discipline is a Mark of Sonship

I've spent a lot of time in this first part peeling away the layers of deception surrounding willful participation with sin (especially that of pornography) because I want you to see it for what it is. As we wrap up this first part, I want to leave you with what you can do right now to begin walking free. If you're already free, these things are key to staying free.

First realize that confession is a vital part of becoming and staying free. You must admit to yourself and to God what evil thoughts and desires you've given your love and attention. State plainly before the Father what you've participated with, who you've hurt (including yourself), and what you've done. Don't try to cloak or disguise it. He already knows anyway. But He does not condemn us. First John 1:9 says He is faithful and just both to forgive us ALL sins and cleanse us of ALL unrighteousness. All means all. He can and will cleanse us and give us new life.

Secondly, you must repent. Unfortunately for many, repentance carries a negative connotation, especially when it is not properly understood. However, a biblical understanding of repentance makes it both very practical and desirable. For starters, to repent simply means to turn and go a different direction. Why would we want to continue heading down a road we know leads to destruction? So we turn around and pursue life through Jesus and by the guiding of the Holy Spirit. It is simple and powerful, but it does require submission. Part of repentance is that we obey the Lord and not ourselves or our desires.

Nevertheless, it is important to understand that repentance is actually a gift. We cannot accomplish it on our own, but the grace of God empowers us to live it out. Repentance actually transforms the way someone thinks. As a person turns from their sin and begins to focus on hearing and obeying God, the Holy Spirit reveals God's way of thinking. The old understanding passes away, replaced by a new, more powerful way of living. All of this comes about by God's goodness toward us. Romans 2:4 says that it is God's goodness that leads us to repentance. One way of looking at it is this: if God's goodness is leading me to repentance, then my job is to submit to and follow after the goodness of God to me. He wants me to have this gift, and if I follow Him, I will have it. Once I've received this great gift, it will transform not only how I act, but how I think.

That's an empowering way of seeing repentance. Yes, we still must choose, but when we see it as a function of God's goodness, it is easy to choose repentance over those old thoughts and actions.

Finally, I encourage you to embrace the discipline of God. Hebrews 12: 3-11 describes God's discipline beautifully: "For consider Him who endured such hostility from sinners against Himself, lest you become weary and discouraged in your souls. You have not yet resisted to bloodshed, striving against sin. And you have forgotten the exhortation which speaks to you as to sons: 'My son, do not despise the chastening of the Lord, Nor be discouraged when you are rebuked by Him; For whom the Lord loves He chastens, And scourges every son whom He receives.' If you endure chastening, God deals with you as with sons; for what son is there whom a father does not chasten? But if you are without chastening, of which all have become partakers, then you are illegitimate and not sons. Furthermore, we have had human fathers who corrected us, and we paid them respect. Shall we not much more readily be in subjection to the Father of spirits and live? For they indeed for a few days chastened us as seemed best to them, but He for our profit, that we may be partakers of His holiness. Now no chastening seems to be joyful for the present, but painful; nevertheless, afterward it yields the peaceable fruit of righteousness to those who have been trained by it."

God's discipline may take different forms, but the important thing is to ask Him for His discipline and obey what He shows you. You may confess to those you've hurt and ask forgiveness. You may sit out from ministry for a while and seek His face. You may fast, go on a retreat to be with Him, or step down from some position. God knows exactly what we need. Remember, too, that His purpose is to train us, restore us, and produce righteousness in us. It's not about punishment; it's about living in His holiness.

I would encourage you to seek guidance from those who have spiritual authority in your life. Share your heart and invite your pastor or spiritual head to walk this out with you. That will protect you from punishing yourself unduly, and it will also help you discern the will of the Lord. At the very least, I would recommend sharing this journey with mature believers who can love you through the process.

However all of this looks for you, I know you'll be blessed in walking in the discipline of the Lord. After all, God could have simply given us over to those evil desires and the destruction that follows (Romans 1:28-32). Instead, He has chosen to correct us as His beloved children. That way, He can lead us into the magnificent plans He has for us.

In the next part, we will look at some specifics of how temptation works and how Jesus has blessed us to overcome in every area. Before you read on, however, I encourage you to pray through any confession and repentance you feel led to pray. Then worship the Lord for His goodness to you, and ask Him to correct you and discipline you as a son. Finally, ask Him to fill you afresh with His unfailing love.

He really does love us.

LIBERATED

PART TWO: BLESSED TO ENDURE

As Christians, we have been blessed with the nature of Jesus Christ. True, the Holy Spirit continues to prune us and develop the nature of our Lord throughout our lives. None of us have fully attained to it yet, but the fact remains, we have been blessed with the mind of Christ, as well as an increasing portion of His nature (1 Corinthians 2:16 and 2 Peter 1:2-4).

One of Jesus's most important characteristics is that He overcame every single obstacle thrown at Him. He conquered and destroyed all the weakness inherent in fallen mankind, He withstood and defeated every temptation known to man, and ultimately, He tore down the curtain of separation that kept us from the Father's very presence.

In short, He endured to the end, and He was victorious.

Jesus is also building His endurance in us. He calls His people to overcome temptation and sin the same way He did. Our own strength cannot push us to victory, but His Spirit empowers us to overcome. Just as Jesus lived in full submission to the Father, we must fully submit to the Spirit, agreeing with what His Word says about us and obeying what He says on a minute-by-minute basis. It isn't always easy, but it is simple.

In this section, we'll look at what it really means to *endure*, specifically what it means to endure temptation. We'll examine what's happening when we feel overwhelmed by temptation and the desire to sin, along with some of the most simple and powerful ways to render that attack powerless. Finally, we'll dig into the call to be vigilant against the tricks and snares of the devil.

We are not ignorant of the devices Satan uses to try to destroy us. We may have given in to them in the past, but Jesus is empowering us to ensure that it never happens again. Complete freedom is a possibility, and it starts with simply believing what He has already taught us in His Word.

To Endure is to Overcome

I think it's a misconception to take the Biblical word "endure" as if it just means, "to go through something." It's easy to see why some would understand it this way, since we all go through a great many trials in this life. But when we take into account the word's definition and the context of its use in the Bible, it becomes apparent that to endure means more than just to go through trials or temptations.

We'll start by looking at Jesus as the model of endurance. At the Garden Gathering, our Pastor and Apostle Brandy Helton has taught repeatedly that Jesus is our model in all things. It only makes sense that we should look at Him as our example for how to endure (overcome) temptation.

Start in Hebrews 12:1-2, which says, "Therefore we also, since we are surrounded by so great a cloud of witnesses, let us lay aside every weight, and the sin which so easily ensnares us, and let us run with endurance the race that is set before us, looking unto Jesus, the author and finisher of our faith, who for the joy that was set before Him *endured the cross*, despising the shame, and has sat down at the right hand of the throne of God [emphasis added]."

This passage not only instructs us to lay aside sin (which, as we previously discussed, means there is grace and empowerment to do so), but it also describes Jesus as having endured the cross. Now think about that. What Jesus went through on the cross was terrible beyond imagination! And remember, the physical suffering was not even half the equation. What Jesus suffered in the spiritual realm was far worse than that.

But now ask yourself this question: did the cross win, or did Jesus? Obviously Jesus won. He overcame the cross because

He now sits at the Father's right hand in the heavenly places (Ephesians 1:20-21). The cross did not defeat our Lord. He endured it and is now seated in a place of honor. So from this, you begin to see that to endure is not merely to suffer.

There are more examples. Matthew 4:1-11 documents Jesus's temptation at the hands of Satan. Satan throws some of his best enticements at Jesus, and Jesus completely defeats him. The Lord simply would not allow Satan to move Him from His God-given mission. He refuted the devil with the Word of God, and even when Satan tried to twist Scripture, Jesus did not take the bait. The Lord's final answer was, "You shall worship the Lord your God, and Him only shall you serve." That final counter to the devil's attempts at seduction shows how Jesus overcame: His eyes and His heart were fixed on the Father.

> **WEAPONS OF OUR WARFARE:**
>
> *John 14:12 says, "most assuredly, I say to you, he who believes in Me, the works that I do he will do also; and greater works than these he will do, because I go to My Father." This is Jesus's personal guarantee that He empowers us to walk in His freedom.*

Now remember that, naturally speaking, Jesus was not at His strongest when this exchange took place. He'd just been baptized in water and the Holy Spirit and was led immediately into the wilderness, where He fasted for forty days. I imagine He felt gnawing hunger pain. He was probably covered head to toe in dust. He faced the dangers and hardships of living in the wilderness, all while completely isolated. And yet, even in what would appear as a weak moment, Jesus *endured*. He overcame what Satan threw at Him, and overwhelmingly defeated the enemy.

Another Scripture, Hebrews 4:15-16, tells us that Jesus was tempted in *all points* just like we are, yet He did not sin. In other words, there's nothing you could say to Jesus about what Satan uses to tempt you that He couldn't reply, "He tried that on me too." And still, Jesus endured.

Finally, James 1:12 says, "Blessed is the man who endures temptation; for when he has been approved, he will receive the crown of life which the Lord has promised to those who love Him." This passage makes it apparent that enduring temptation results in being approved and receiving the crown of life. Would someone who simply suffered from temptation and gave into it be approved and receive a crown? I think you get the point. I'd also like to suggest that this passage connects loving the Lord to endurance. Jesus overcame temptation because of His great love for the Father, which He demonstrated through His complete submission. In the same way, one major part of endurance is to stay focused on the love Jesus has for us, and the love we have for Him.

To continue, though, you can see that in all these passages, the word "endure" suggests not only suffering from or passing through a trial or temptation, but overcoming it by the Spirit. Strong's concordance sheds even more light on the meaning of this word.

The word used in James 1 is Strong's number 5278: hupomeno. It means "*to stay under (behind), i.e. remain; figuratively to undergo, i.e. bear (trials), have fortitude, persevere.*" So you see that while the word's literal meaning is to undergo or remain in something, its extended meaning includes fortitude and perseverance. **From the life of Jesus and the Scriptures we've been looking at, it is clear that God's intent is not merely for us to go through temptation but to overcome it.**

Some people reading this may think, "Well that was Jesus, and I'm not Him."

However, while Jesus was still fully God as He walked this earth, He emptied Himself of that position and lived as a man in full submission to God. In other words, whatever He did, He did as one of us. And He also promised in John 14:12 that we could do the works He did. We are called, commanded, and blessed to endure, and there are no excuses. If we run with endurance, we will finish the race.

As I've said before, when God commands or calls us to do something, He provides the grace necessary to obey. Scripture makes it clear that God has blessed us to endure (which from now on, will read *overcome, conquer, defeat, etc.*) temptation.

One major step believers can take in overcoming deception and breaking free from bondage is to accept what Scripture has already told us about ourselves. Many people see defeating temptation as a pre-requisite to being blessed, but the truth is we are already blessed. Notice that the passage above from James chapter 1 doesn't say, "Blessed will you eventually be when you finally manage to overcome temptation." It says, "Blessed IS the man who endures temptation..."[emphasis added]. In other words, the blessing to overcome is in effect right this minute, not in some unspecified time in the future.

Also, remember that 2 Peter 1:2-4 says we've been given all things that pertain to life and godliness. Not only that, but the promises we have received empower us to partake of God's nature and to escape corruption. These are promises we *have received*, meaning they're in our possession and available for our immediate use.

Furthermore, Ephesians 1:3-4 says, "Blessed be the God and Father of our Lord Jesus Christ, who has blessed us with every spiritual blessing in the heavenly places in Christ, just as He chose us in Him before the foundation of the world, that we should be holy and without blame before Him in love." We have been blessed with every spiritual blessing. That means the blessing to endure is ours, and the time to put it to work is right now!

What I'm hoping you are starting to see is that to live a sin-free life by the grace and power of the Holy Spirit is actually a possibility! Jesus modeled it for us, and the keys for Him were the same keys for us: love and obedience. And like He said, if He did it, we can do it.

An important step is to reject the mindset that you're a sinner and receive the new identity Jesus bought for you: a righteous son. Romans 5:18-19 says, "Therefore, as through one man's offense judgment came to all men, resulting in condemnation, even so through one Man's righteous act the free gift came to all men, resulting in justification of life. For as by one man's disobedience many were made sinners, so also by one Man's obedience many will be made righteous." Jesus has made us righteous as a matter of position with the Father, and He has also given us His blessing to live in perfect righteousness in practice. Again, if He said it, that means we can do it.

Yes, I'm well aware that none of us are there yet, but we must renew our minds to see the truth that we can start overcoming bondage and crushing temptation right now. **As long as we continue to think of ourselves as sinners, we will continue to sin. As long as we see the power of temptation to drag us down as greater than the power of the cross to set us free, we'll continue to lose.** That's not what I want, and it is certainly not what the Father wants for us.

A good starting place in renewing our minds is to recognize one of Satan's most vicious and sneaky lies, which is the mentality, "I will always struggle with this." We need to destroy that way of thinking in order to walk in victory over sin.

It is true that we will have to make some effort, and it is likely that we will have to make some changes. It may not always be easy. But it is possible. To resign ourselves to a lifetime of struggle against the same temptation is to deny the power of the sacrifice Jesus made and to reject what His Word says about who we truly are. If He says we can be free, then we can be free. Period.

It's time we started thinking that way.

The Bombardment

I know from experience, and have had this confirmed many times over in conversations I've had with others struggling with temptations and bondage, that sometimes, temptation feels like a war. There's even a mindset I've dealt with in myself and others that runs something like this: "I'll be good for a time. I'll be strong. But something happens, I see something, or I just start getting complacent. And then it's just a matter of time until I get worn down and give in to that sin."

In my past, I have felt that I had to be 100% at all times, and if I ever got tired, angry, frustrated, or simply a little down, then I was in serious danger of stepping back into sin. It even fostered a mindset in me that agreed with the notion that sooner or later, regardless of how hard I tried, I would eventually fail.

One week. One month. Half a year. Boom! Right back in it again. Which basically made me feel like a total failure. That is really just part of what Satan is trying to accomplish in the first place. Remember that the enemy ultimately wants to shut us down and stop us short of our God-given destiny. That's the desired end-game any time the enemy is involved.

As I allowed the Lord to teach me about why walking in freedom from porn always seemed like an uphill battle, He gave me revelation that the enemy really does approach temptation like a siege situation.

Imagine the old days when an army would march up to a walled city, surround it, and set in for the long haul. A cunning commander would not immediately rush up to the walled fortress and try to take it down. That would be a sure way to lose a lot of troops and not accomplish much. As long as the people in that walled city were fresh, well-fed, well-rested, and well-supplied, they made for a near-unbeatable foe.

So the strategy was to wait. Cut off all supply lines. Let time and frustrations take their toll. Hurl taunts and insults at the opponent, baiting them into making brash and ill-advised choices. Wear them down to the point that weaknesses revealed themselves. Then attack full-force.

That's just like what the devil does to people struggling with addiction. He doesn't attack straightforwardly. He

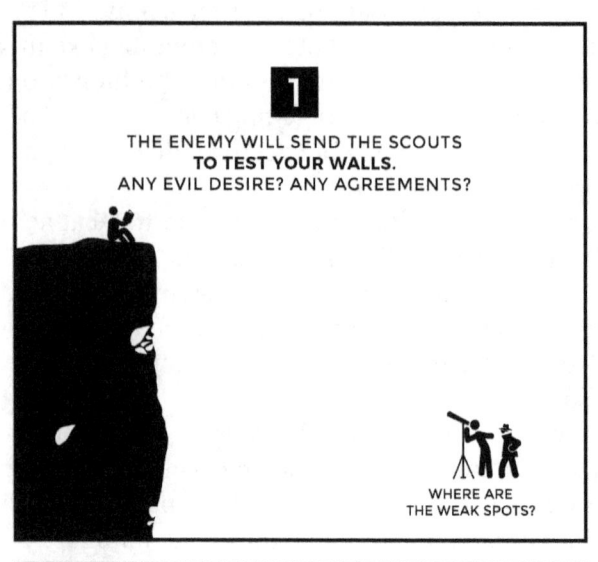

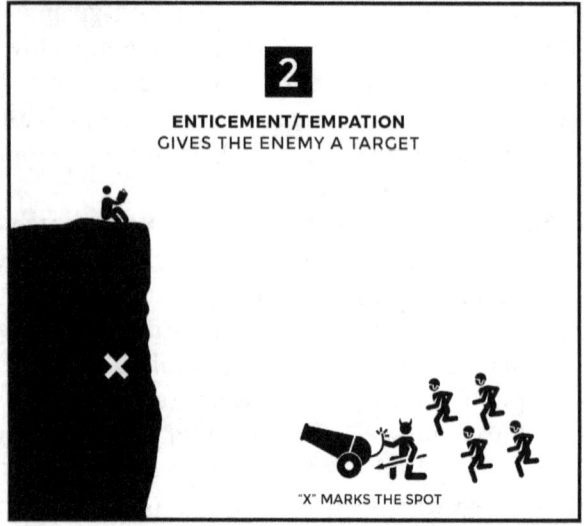

1

THE ENEMY WILL SEND THE SCOUTS **TO TEST YOUR WALLS**.
ANY EVIL DESIRE? ANY AGREEMENTS?

WHERE ARE THE WEAK SPOTS?

2

ENTICEMENT/TEMPATION
GIVES THE ENEMY A TARGET

"X" MARKS THE SPOT

waits for the opportune time. He shoots the arrows of ungodly thoughts. He questions us relentlessly. He throws shame and guilt at us. He tries to isolate us from those who strengthen us. If we make a false move, he attacks.

This basic strategy is no secret. I teach high school

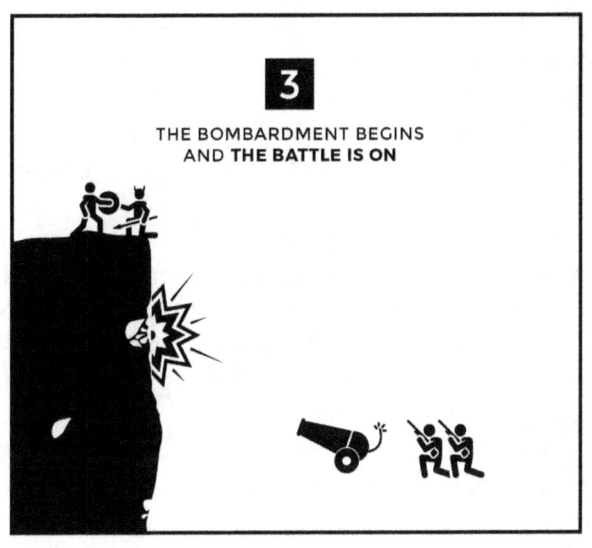

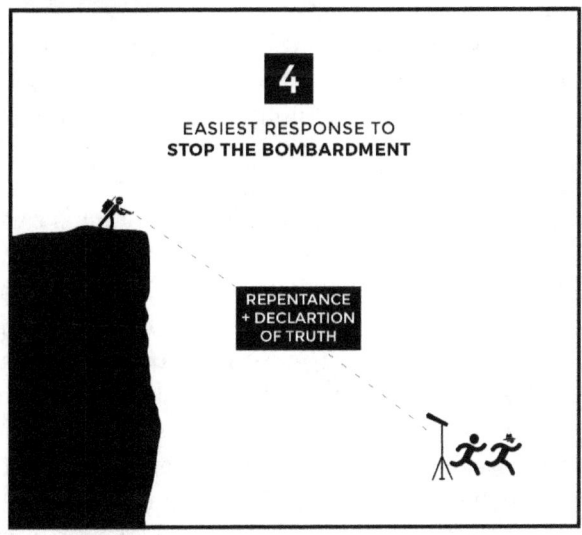

3

THE BOMBARDMENT BEGINS
AND **THE BATTLE IS ON**

4

EASIEST RESPONSE TO
STOP THE BOMBARDMENT

REPENTANCE
+ DECLARTION
OF TRUTH

English for a living, and even I can see the effectiveness of these tactics for taking down a walled city. The Bible says we are not ignorant of the devices of Satan, so there is really no mystery to this kind of attack.

But our enemy keeps doing this because it keeps working.

So let's take it back to James 1 and look at why this tactic is still so effective despite its overwhelming simplicity. James 1:13-15 tells us, "Let no one say when he is tempted, 'I am tempted by God'; for God cannot be tempted by evil, nor does He Himself tempt anyone. But each one is tempted when he is drawn away by his own desires and enticed. Then, when desire has conceived, it gives birth to sin, and sin, when it is full-grown, brings forth death."

Once again, we see the pattern clearly: enticement-drawn away-temptation-sin-death. I keep emphasizing the "death" part because I want you to see this in its most serious terms: the enemy is out to kill you. He will set a siege around your walls, and if he breaks through your defenses, he will slaughter you without mercy.

To get really practical with this, I want to describe this onslaught, this bombardment, in such a way that you see the strategy involved, as well as the countermoves that will defeat this tactic of the enemy.

For starters, God showed me that, while the enemy is really stupid in a lot of ways, he is not a fool when it comes to strategy. He uses maneuvers that work. Ever notice that the devil doesn't attack you in places where you're strong? That would be really poor battle strategy.

Imagine an ancient commander setting up his catapults and launching stones at the strongest part of a wall. What a magnificent waste of time that would be! The better strategy is to find the parts of the wall that are not as strong and launch the attack there. **The bombardment is meant to take an already weak area and create an opening for the real attack to break through.**

In similar fashion, Satan's temptations will come at us in places where he thinks he can win. Is there some kind of evil desire lurking within us? Is there any agreement in our mind or heart that he can exploit? Is there any unforgiveness? Is there some kind of sin in operation, or that has not been repented of? That's where the bombardment will come.

In my own experience, the bombardment comes in the form of a thought-barrage. It can be memories of videos I've seen or watched, fantasies, what-if scenarios, even dreams at night. I've literally spent entire days shooing off what felt like a swarm of flies in the form of all these kinds of thoughts. So what's the goal? Entice me. Get my attention. Draw me off. Get me to agree or participate. Breach my wall.

> **◆ WEAPONS OF OUR WARFARE:**
>
> *Prayer of Faith. The prayers in this section will have as much power as you have faith in what the Lord will do. It is pointless to simply say words. Put your trust in what Jesus said, that if we ask and do not doubt, it will be done for us.*

As God taught me about how this type of attack works, He also showed me how to use the enemy's strategy against him. It's really simple: **I cannot be enticed by something that does not have my attention.** Just like the person sitting outside the bakery I described in part one, I will only be tempted to eat cookies if I am aware they exist. If the cookies represent sinful thoughts or behaviors, my choice then becomes whether or not to stay in a place where I know temptation lives. Or, I can choose to feast on healthy foods rather than eating cookies.

Spiritually speaking, I have power to decide what I give my attention to, and if Jesus occupies my mind, there's no room for other thoughts to have any power. Think of your mind like a vessel. If that vessel is completely full of pure water, there is no room for anything else to come in. Even if ungodly thoughts or desires do start to get my attention, I've been given power and authority to destroy ungodly thoughts. I simply place myself beneath the pure stream again and allow it to purge whatever came in.

Likewise, I cannot be drawn away by something that I do

not desire. I dare you to try to draw me away by tempting me to go get a tooth pulled. It won't work. Temptations can only draw us if we actually desire them. If I find myself being tempted, the response is to search out my heart, find what desire is in operation, and allow Jesus to destroy it.

Here's where it gets even more freeing: if I feel something knocking on my door, some thought or memory or whatever trying out its chisel to test the strength of my wall, I need to do what the archers of old would do and shoot it down immediately. The Bible says we can take our thoughts captive to the obedience of Christ (2 Corinthians 10:5). Simply refuse to give those thoughts your attention in the first place. And if they persist, shoot them. Take them captive in Jesus' name. Cast them down to be destroyed. You'll notice that the scouts quit coming when they keep getting shot.

Practically, you can pray like this: "Father, in the name of Jesus, I renounce and rebuke the ungodly thoughts coming my way. I take them captive to the obedience of Jesus Christ. In Jesus' name I rebuke the source of those thoughts and I command them to be captured and bound in the name of Jesus. I charge the angels assigned to me to take those evil spirits where Jesus has sent them never to return, in the name of Jesus, and I thank You Father for turning my thoughts to righteousness. Amen."

If you're praying this way, but the thoughts and temptations keep coming, that tells you there's a deeper reason for it. Remember, the enemy is not going to attack you somewhere unless he thinks he can win there. So what's making him think he has a shot at you? Very likely, there is an evil desire in your heart that he's trying to exploit. Or there is an ungodly agreement you've made with something not of God. Or possibly, you've started to actively participate with the enemy through your continued entertainment of ungodly thinking or actions. The bombardment has begun.

Fortunately, there is a remedy called repentance. Repentance and the accompanying forgiveness we receive bring in the reinforcements of Heaven. If the wall was weak ten seconds ago, repentance makes it strong again, so long as the repentance comes from the heart.

Too many times a believer will pray a prayer of verbal repentance without actually allowing the Lord to destroy the desire or the agreement that is in operation in his heart. I cannot count the number of times I prayed through repentance because I felt guilty and not because I seriously wanted to kill the evil desire in operation in my heart. My friends, that kind of prayer is not warfare – it's just a delay.

Why do we pray when we have no intention of allowing the desire to die? Part of the equation is pleasure. The pleasure we take from whatever we're desiring lays hold in our flesh, and if it continues long enough, we give our hearts to it as well. In the *Iliad*, the Greeks disguised an invasion force by building what appeared to be a peace offering. The Trojan Horse, as we know it, would have remained a harmless and ineffective piece of junk had the Trojans left it outside the gate. However, in their pride, the Trojans brought the Trojan Horse inside their city, inviting in the very force that would destroy them.

In similar fashion, the pleasure we derive from ungodly thoughts or actions can disguise an enemy as something desirable, tempting us to allow it inside our hearts. Once that happens, we must either kill the invaders, or they will methodically take us down. Allowing the Lord to pluck out and destroy the pleasure we have taken from ungodly desire is a necessary part of freedom.

We have to allow the Lord to search us and know us and reveal if there is any wickedness at work in us (Psalm 139:23). Then, from our heart, we allow Him to destroy the evil things in operation and to fill us with His goodness and love. That is what makes real repentance possible, and that will make your wall strong.

Again, you can pray like this: "Father, in the name of Jesus, I confess that I have taken pleasure in _____. I ask You to forgive me and cleanse me according to Your Word. I renounce all pleasure I have taken from ____ in the name of Jesus, and I give You permission to pluck it up from my heart and destroy it. I decree that this pleasure is dead and that it may not return in Jesus name. In the name of Jesus, I renounce every evil desire connected to this pleasure and I destroy it by the blood of Jesus Christ. Lord, I ask You to fill me with Your goodness and mercy, along with Your love, and I thank You for it."

When you find yourself in the midst of the onslaught, you must get really honest with yourself and before God. Allow the Holy Spirit to reveal to you where the beginning of this battle truly lies. Then repent. Renounce your desire and your participation with every form of evil. Do not fall into the trap of thinking that you dealt with a certain sin before, so it shouldn't be operating now. Repent again! Then receive your forgiveness and your healing by faith. Don't forget to forgive yourself. You're rebuilding your wall with the Master Builder, so let no stone remain out of place.

Let me pause for a moment and say this: I am not teaching you to focus on what Satan is trying to do in your life and use that as your basis for operation. As always, Jesus is the one we look to in our daily lives. However, I am teaching that we must recognize when an enemy scout shows up on our doorstep in the form of temptation. That should be the first hint that we need to allow the Holy Spirit to search us and reveal why that scout has come. Furthermore, if the enemy ramps up the attack with more bombardment, we must acknowledge that there is a reason for that and run to the Lord in repentance. Ignoring an enemy force will inevitably lead to defeat. The wiser choice is to take immediate and overwhelming action.

Ultimately, our best chance at victory is to see the enemy army from a long way off and allow the host of Heaven to deal with it before it gets to our doorstep. That's why Hebrews 12:2 exhorts us to focus on Jesus, the author and finisher of our faith. He can tell us when there's danger, and if we listen to Him, that enemy army will never get close enough to attack.

One final note on the practical side of this battle: one of the best weapons you have in your arsenal is to be transparent with those the Lord has called you to walk alongside. I encourage you to open up with your spouse, your trusted friends, your pastor, or anyone the Holy Spirit leads you to do so with any time you feel yourself being enticed or drawn. Don't wait until the situation becomes critical before you take action. Even then, you can still win the fight, but the best policy is to cut temptation off before it has a chance to produce any fruit in the first place.

How silly would it be for one of those soldiers of old to see a weak spot in the wall and try to hide it? That would basically guarantee that the enemy had a place available for attack! And yet, that's exactly what a lot of us do when we start to notice the enticement taking place. Instead of shooting down that spy with the chisel, we pretend it's not there.

I can't tell anybody this is what I'm feeling. They'll think I sinned already. I prayed over this already. It's not really there; I'm just overcoming again. I'll be embarrassed to admit that this is happening yet again. What if they don't understand? What if I lose my position?

I have experienced every one of those thoughts, and regrettably, I've submitted to them out of fear of being exposed, fear of rejection, fear of losing respect, and just plain old pride. And I've left myself vulnerable to attack.

One of the biggest breakthroughs I've ever experienced was finally choosing to open up with my wife when I felt the enticement coming. Rather than allowing that hook to set in, I brought what I was experiencing into the light, where it lost its power. Furthermore, the anointed prayers of my wife annihilated what I was dealing with, and we both felt protected in the process.

If you're single, you can get the same level of freedom by opening with a brother, sister, pastor, or someone you trust. Get their agreement working for you, and shine the light on that weak spot. Allow those the Lord has positioned to walk with you to speak life and encouragement to you, and build up your wall again.

Ephesians 5:13-14 speaks to the power of bringing temptation to light: "But all things that are exposed are made manifest by the light, for whatever makes manifest is light. Therefore He says: 'Awake, you who sleep, Arise from the dead, And Christ will give you light.'" The light of Jesus makes it clear where and what our enemy is.

Finally, John 3:18-21 says, "He who believes in Him is not condemned; but he who does not believe is condemned already, because he has not believed in the name of the only begotten Son of God. And this is the condemnation, that the light has come into the world, and men loved darkness rather than light, because their deeds were evil. For everyone practicing evil hates the light and does not come to the light, lest his deeds should be exposed. But he who does the truth comes to the light, that his deeds may be clearly seen, that they have been done in God." Here, Jesus teaches that those who belong to God bring their deeds into the light that they may be clearly seen. We choose to live in the truth. The enemy will try everything he can to keep you agreeing with him, hiding in the darkness.

The Light of God that exposes darkness also has the power to destroy darkness.

Lastly, if you're actively watching, praying, and maintaining openness before the Lord, yet you still feel like you're struggling, that is a clear sign that it is time for you to get some deliverance. Do not delay in setting up a time of prayer so that the Lord can go deep with you and set you free from the demonic power at work.

This battle is one we can win every time. If we're honest with ourselves and before the Lord about what is going on inside us, if we allow Him to search us out and destroy evil desires, and if we refuse to give our attention to the darkness, we make our walls strong. Even during times of attack, we can repent and receive forgiveness, and thereby turn the tide of the battle back in our favor. Finally, we can choose to live our lives out in the open, in the light, which makes it awfully hard for the enemy to sneak up on us in the first place.

Be Vigilant!

The Lord wants us to win. He gave us a blessing of endurance, and He remains for us in the presence of the Father as a merciful and faithful high priest. He has clearly exposed the schemes of the enemy and has given us weapons to overcome. All that is required for us to live in victory has been made available through the Lord Jesus.

The one part of the equation that tends to be missing is our part, which is to be vigilant. First Peter 5:8-11 makes our role clear: "Be sober, be vigilant; because your adversary the devil walks about like a roaring lion, seeking whom he may devour. Resist him, steadfast in the faith, knowing that the same sufferings are experienced by your brotherhood in the world. But may the God of all grace, who called us to His eternal glory by Christ Jesus, after you have suffered a while, perfect, establish, strengthen, and settle you. To Him be the glory and the dominion forever and ever. Amen."

This familiar passage makes it clear that the believer must remain sober-minded and vigilant. It also commands (and therefore blesses) us to resist the devil, steadfast in our faith in Jesus. We are blessed to stand fast and not be moved by Satan's tricks and temptations. But we still must choose to whom we submit, which requires our spiritual alertness and quick obedience to Holy Spirit.

Part of being sober and vigilant is to recognize when we are vulnerable to attack. As I've said already, Satan understands sound strategy, so he tends to attack not only areas of weakness, but also at opportune times. Think about when you've felt the most attacked or tempted. I'm betting if you mapped those times out, there was some kind of emotional background going on that further sapped your will to defend your wall or made you less aware of what was going on. It's almost like a smoke screen meant to disguise the true attack.

Here are some times that vigilance is especially vital:
- After you've been angry
- During times of sadness or disappointment
- When you've felt rejected by your spouse, friends, or colleagues
- When you're mentally or physically tired
- When you've been busy – especially much busier than you normally are
- After some kind of conflict with those close to you
- When you're under a lot of stress

Now, I'm not a psychologist or counselor, but I have experienced these feelings and situations myself. Probably none of the items on the list so far are surprising to you. All of these emotions and circumstances are unpleasant, to say the least, and they put us into an emotional state that makes our souls vulnerable to attack. These are the times when the attack may not even seem like an attack, or, silly as it sounds, when we can see the attack but choose not to take action because of all the other issues going on.

Nevertheless, the Bible's command to remain vigilant is vital because that vigilance is what keeps the wall protected and safe. I'd liken this to a watchman failing to sound the alarm at the sight of the enemy because the watchman had a busy week and just felt too tired to do anything. That makes no sense whatsoever, and obviously that watchman will be held accountable for his actions (or lack thereof).

Another insidious part of the attack is that, during these times of emotional turmoil, the sin likes to pose as Holy Spirit. It comes as a false comforter, offering a sense of release, a sense of power, or even a temporary pleasure in the midst of the turmoil. So many times, that's why we let the gate down and invite the sin in. Deception! We must remain vigilant and open-eyed especially in emotionally demanding situations.

The Holy Spirit will warn us and correct us, but we must choose to listen and obey. Furthermore, we must choose in that moment to listen to the truth and not seek out some false comfort in the arms of the assassin. As you know, that does not end well. But the passage above encourages us to remain steadfast in the faith, knowing that the reward for doing so is that Jesus Himself will perfect, establish, strengthen, and settle us. We receive these blessings as we overcome, so take heart!

It may surprise you, however, that it is not only during the emotionally hard times that Satan finds opportunity to attack. One of the times we can be most vulnerable is during what we might describe as "spiritual highs" – those times we're feeling strong or when something great has been happening in our spiritual walk. Just like the Trojans in the old story, we can sometimes get so caught up in the celebration that we unwittingly invite a destructive attack. We let our guard down, so to speak, and the enemy finds his opening.

As the Holy Spirit was teaching me this, He took me to Luke 17:5-10: "And the apostles said to the Lord, "Increase our faith." So the Lord said, "If you have faith as a mustard seed, you can say to this mulberry tree, 'Be pulled up by the roots and be planted in the sea,' and it would obey you. And which of you, having a servant plowing or tending sheep, will say to him when he has come in from the field, 'Come at once and sit down to eat'? But will he not rather say to him, 'Prepare something for my supper, and gird yourself and serve me till I have eaten and drunk, and afterward you will eat and drink'? Does he thank that servant because he did the things that were commanded him? I think not. So likewise you, when you have done all those things which you are commanded, say, 'We are unprofitable servants. We have done what was our duty to do.'"

This passage is rich with application to a number of areas, but I want to focus in on what Jesus is teaching them about the aftermath of the spiritual highs. The apostles wanted an increase of faith, and I believe Jesus showed them exactly how to get it. But before He did that, the Lord pointed out that it was not the *amount* of faith they had that truly mattered, since a mustard seed's worth could perform such amazing miracles. For the sake of the topic we're exploring, if you've felt that you're struggling because you don't have enough faith, let this passage destroy that mindset.

But to continue, Jesus showed the disciples how a servant would go and do his work, then return to the house and *serve the master*. He is trying to change their viewpoint away from that of coming back in to be served, and toward that of coming in to the house to serve the One through whom the power to work was given. And the Lord emphasizes His point by telling them that after they had done those things they were commanded (which for a believer includes signs, miracles, and wonders), they should view that as simply their duty.

When I see a miracle, it fires me up. I get so excited about it that it stays with me for days. Whether it's a healing, a deliverance, or some other awesome work, I can't help being "spiritually high." I'm not even saying that's necessarily a bad thing, but I'm drawing attention to one area of vigilance that Jesus brought up: as believers, we should expect the amazing manifestations of the Kingdom of Heaven as a normal part of our lives. It's not that we should dismiss those manifestations of His goodness or refuse to be excited about them. However, Jesus is basically saying, "My friends, this is business as usual for us, so don't let these things steal so much of your attention that you lose focus on Me."

How many times have you come back from a conference or event completely amped up, only to find yourself in the following days and weeks struggling or even participating with sin? Or how many times has some awesome thing the Lord did in your life caused you to let your focus drift backwards to that event instead of keeping your eyes focused forward and on Him?

Part of what Jesus is showing us is that after we do our work as His servants, we ought to remain vigilant and humble by immediately serving Him. It's not time to rest on what may seem like our accomplishment, but rather to serve the Lord. We serve Him in our worship, in our intimacy with Him, and by keeping our eyes fixed on Him. That puts Jesus in His rightful place in our hearts. The spiritual high becomes a normal part of our experience, and we are not as vulnerable anymore because we are intently focused on the true source of our strength! (For what it's worth, that's also how we increase our faith.)

Our measure of vigilance is basically the degree to which we continue to focus on Jesus, regardless of the high or low state we happen to be in. And it's not supposed to be hard. Jesus is our friend, our hero, our inspiration, our priest, and our advocate. He's on our side. He's our biggest ally and our most ferocious defender. Coming to Him and focusing on Him are part of our normal life, but that simple act of focus makes such a huge difference.

Many who are genuine believers honestly think they can never be free. "If I'm still fighting and having to keep my guard up," the reasoning goes, "then am I truly free?" The answer is absolutely yes. It just means you sometimes have to make some effort to keep your freedom. Even in the secular world, people repeatedly affirm that freedom isn't free.

> **WEAPONS OF OUR WARFARE:**
>
> ***Choices.*** *Since Satan cannot force saints to act according to his will, we always get to choose. God provides the way out. When we choose to follow God's way, deliberately and with determination, we effectively resist the devil. It is dangerous to postpone the choice. A friend of mine is fond of telling her kids, "Obey, right away, without delay." That saying applies in these situations as well.*

Our freedom cost Jesus dearly, but He has bought and paid for it in full. It is ours! And just as in the world maintaining freedom often requires action, spiritual freedom requires a continual submission to the Holy Spirit. Remember that the onslaught will usually happen when Satan thinks he has a chance to win. The other times of enticement are just spies with chisels and are easily dealt with. In both cases, we're well-equipped to defeat the attack.

Take courage and choose to believe in the freedom that

Jesus purchased at the cross. Freedom does not mean that we will always have to fight, but it does require that we remain vigilant and focused on the source of our freedom – Jesus.

He was tempted so He could destroy the power of temptation. He was destroyed so that we can be restored. He endured to the end so that He could freely give to us His blessing to endure!

PART THREE: STAND FAST

From my own past with pornography, I can attest that believers sometimes have a tendency to live in cycles. The spiritual highs give way to a downward turn toward apathy. Apathy turns into temptation, leading to sin. Sin produces its fruit of death in its many forms, such as depression, relationships suffering, or simply turning away from God. Then God, in His mercy and grace, draws us out of that hole and back toward Him. The cycle repeats.

That was pretty much my life story from the time I got saved at the age of seventeen until about ten years later when I finally accepted God's invitation to end the cycle. It's not that I wasn't growing spiritually during those years or that sin was the overarching characteristic of my life, but sin was definitely a major ongoing issue, and it definitely hindered my advancement in the Kingdom.

You see, the cycle I was stuck in (or rather, willingly chose to live in) kept me from truly wanting to press forward in the Kingdom. Doing so would mean I'd have to give up my false lover, my crutch that I ran to for so many reasons. I honestly didn't know what life would look like without pornography or masturbation, since I had lived with them since I was twelve. Furthermore, I was unwilling to be around believers who were passionately pursuing Jesus, since they made me feel so shallow and filthy by comparison. And ultimately, I dreaded being in a room with prophetic people because I was constantly afraid of being called out and humiliated.

So I was stuck and I stayed stuck.

But God!

As God led me out of the cycle that had dominated my life for so many years, He showed me enough of His character that I could finally trust that humiliation was never His goal for me. His prophets would speak to me the same way He does: with firm correction but gentle encouragement as well. And the Holy Spirit testified to me about the power of the cross, showing me that Jesus didn't die to leave us in our sin. When Jesus said, "It is finished," He meant it. That meant remaining stuck in cycles was really not an option for those who believe in Him.

As I laid hold of my true identity as saint and sanctified one, and let go of the old identity of sinner, I experienced a new level of freedom from fear and cycles. I feared prophetic people less, and I became more willing to imitate the example of the true followers of Jesus.

And yet, there was still a part I had to fulfill with Jesus that nobody else could carry out on my behalf: I had to choose. The reality with pornography, as with most sin, is that we know better than to participate with it. It's not a secret that porn, drugs, alcoholism, overeating, or any form of sin is bad. It is readily apparent to anyone who is willing to be honest about it. But we still choose to step into it. We aren't overcome. It isn't an accident. It's not okay because other people do it. It's not natural. It's not something we need.

It is a choice. We make it. End of story.

While it is true that participation with sin leads to demonic oppression and strongholds being built, the devil has no power to *force* a believer in Jesus to do anything. He cannot possess us because we are bought and paid for by the Blood of Christ! So that tells us that anytime we're in sin, we're there because we made a choice, we made an agreement. Deliverance is a necessary part of any believer's journey, but so is choosing according to the grace of God and not according to the flesh with its desires.

Do not be deceived! Remember that it is possible to live free and clean, whatever that may look like. Along with the blessing to see truth, we have been given another powerful command and blessing: "Stand fast, therefore, in the liberty by which Christ has made us free, and do not be entangled again with a yoke of bondage" (Galatians 5:1).

That's one of the biggest keys to breaking out of the cycle and living free. We must choose to stand fast. We must refuse to be moved. We must submit to God so that the devil flees from us. We must obey the Holy Spirit constantly, by choice, so that the enemy has nowhere to attack us. Our wall must remain strong and grow stronger by the moment as we allow our Friend, Counselor, Guide, and Advocate to lead our lives.

As with most truths in the Kingdom, the reality of standing fast is simple, yet profound. It is not always easy, but it is not complicated either. Our choices must change if our lives are ever to change. There is grace available that makes this possible. Moreover, the love of God, our mightiest weapon, never fails. His love is the final trump card in the game that makes our victory not only possible, but readily available.

This third and final part is both the invitation and the command we have received from our Lord. He purchased our freedom at the cross with His very own blood. Now, with Him at our side and the Holy Ghost as our leader, we must choose His freedom. We must choose to stand fast.

Learn to Distinguish Whose Voice You're Hearing

I know from experience that oftentimes when we step into sin, it can be easy to start agreeing with thoughts like these: *I am a screw-up. I'll probably never break free. I can't keep fighting this battle. I'm just tired of being a loser.*

Some of these lies may even come across as if they were from the Holy Spirit because they seem humble and contrite. The problem is, that shred of humility is mixed with a big dose of lies and self-pity. Furthermore, thinking this way lends itself to remaining stuck in the pit of condemnation. Holy Spirit doesn't work that way. **His conviction is clear and unmistakably direct, but it comes with the empowerment** to change.

You'll start to recognize Holy Spirit talking when you hear the truth spoken in love like this: "You did mess up, and badly, but you are not a screw-up. You're a son. You're a king. You know better, so now is the time to live better. You will never break free in your own strength, but the grace of God will break you free. You can't keep fighting this battle by your own ways. Jesus's blood shed on the cross has already paid for your victory. You can only win by surrendering to Him. Then you won't be tired anymore because you'll be led in triumph."

> **WEAPONS OF OUR WARFARE:**
>
> *Which conversation are you having? Jesus stayed in communion with the Father at all times, and even in temptation, only spoke to the enemy to release the Word of God. Arguing with the enemy is a trap. It is far more powerful to remain in constant conversation with your loving Father and only speak to the enemy as you release what God says toward him. When temptation comes, simply speak to the Lord instead. Try something along these lines: "Father I affirm You as Lord of my life, eternal, and all powerful. Thank You for the revenge You will take on my enemies on my behalf. Your Word says I'm clean because You have spoken to me, and I proclaim my cleanness in Your sight due to the blood of Jesus. Thank You for cleansing and protecting me."*

See the difference? I've learned that Holy Spirit is not afraid to tell me when I'm behaving foolishly, but He never calls me a fool. He does ask me to stop acting like a fool, and He tells me exactly how to do so. Unlike the sly and treacherous voice of condemnation, His voice releases power to change.

When we hear a voice that is not from the Holy Spirit, we must take action quickly. As discussed in Part Two, we can take thoughts captive and cast out the sources of those ungodly thoughts. When we operate that way, it's like flipping on the light in a dark room – which one remains, the darkness or the light? Light always overcomes darkness, but only if we let it shine.

Who Are You, Really?

When Satan tempted Jesus, one of the biggest questions he threw at our Lord was the question of His identity: "If You're really the Son of God, surely You can make bread for Yourself to eat. If He really loves You, You can jump from this high place and God will send His angels to catch You." The derision and mockery are evident here, yet Jesus remained firm in His faith and released His Father's Word. As we've discussed, Jesus was completely victorious.

One key here for those of us desiring to walk in true freedom is that Jesus did not have an identity crisis when the heat was turned up. He was in a forty day period of fasting and temptations, yet He never wavered at the question of who He really was. He knew His God and He knew His purpose. That powerful tool is available to us as well, but it requires a shift in our thinking.

Many times, during periods of temptation, a believer can be deceived into focusing on the negative confession (what I am *not*). We keep telling the devil what we won't do and who we're not going to be, and he keeps coming back with the same kinds of questions he threw at Jesus: "Are you sure you don't want to? Will you really stand strong?"

A more complete and powerful strategy is to stop arguing with the devil and shift our focus upwards. After all, the longer he can keep us engaged, the better chance he has to trip us up or stir an evil desire inside us. While it is unwise to simply ignore the spiritual attack, it is even more unwise to ignore God in the midst of temptation. Where were Jesus's eyes fixed? What was His primary defense? He kept His eyes locked on the Father and His heart full of God's Word. We would do well to imitate that tactic.

First, the best way to really understand our identities

is to allow God to show us who we are to Him. He is our Creator, the author and finisher of our faith. He knows exactly how He designed each one of us to flow and function in union with His Holy Spirit. He can instantly recognize even the tiniest speck that He did not place within us, and He knows exactly how to remove and replace what is not of Him. Gazing into the Father's eyes, we can see our reflection and be encouraged by the way He sees us. His vision and purpose for our lives far outweigh the paltry judgments of the world. His passion overwhelms our short-selling of ourselves. When Satan comes to question and mock, one powerful move we can make is to refuse to give him our full attention and instead, stay focused on the One who loves us beyond measure and who truly gives us our identities.

Second, we can do like Jesus did and speak over ourselves what God's Word says. For example, instead of "I am not a sinful man," our confession becomes, "I am God's handiwork created for good works, which He prepared for me in advance" (Ephesians 2:10). You can take any Scripture that speaks of your identity in Christ and release it verbally. Your spirit will soar as you do this, and the power of that false lover trying to get your attention fades into the backdrop.

I recommend that every person who wants to walk free spend some time prayerfully asking the Holy Spirit to show you the Scriptures that best capture your identity in His eyes. Write them down. Memorize them, and allow them to fill your heart and mind with who you really are. And then, the next time the enemy comes with his sneaky attack, turn to your Father and tell Him how grateful you are that He has made you a son, a priest, a king, an instrument of righteousness, a lover of what is good, a hater of what is evil, His beloved bride...

In light of the siege analogy we discussed in part two, it is vital that we learn to view God as our fortress of strength and our hiding place from the enemy. Psalm 18:2 says, "The Lord is my rock and my fortress and my deliverer; My God, my strength, in whom I will trust; My shield and the horn of my salvation, my stronghold." Keeping our gaze fixed on the Father helps us remain inside His mighty walls of protection and salvation. Allowing Him to reveal our identity and refusing to agree with the lies of the enemy only make the walls of defense even stronger. Then, as we will discuss later, you can launch your own attacks against the enemy.

> **WEAPONS OF OUR WARFARE:**
>
> *Meditate on what is good. Scripture commands followers of Jesus to meditate on what is good, noble, and lovely. This is analogous to filling a container – if my bucket is full of gold, there is no room for someone to put dirt in it. Similarly, if I fill my mind and heart with God's glory and the things of His Kingdom, there's no room for the enemy's filth.*

We Are Led in Triumph

Jesus never intended for any of His saints to live defeated lives. He didn't come and model a life of power, only to show us something we wouldn't receive ourselves. On the contrary, He modeled a completely surrendered life, and He promised that what He did, we would do also (John 14:12).

What was His "secret," His source of power and constant victory? He made it quite clear: "I can of Myself do nothing. As I hear, I judge; and My judgment is righteous, because I do not seek My own will but the will of the Father who sent Me" (John 5:30). Jesus made it clear that the victory and power we are called to carry come from a lifestyle of constant surrender. He did what He saw God doing. He said what He heard God saying. No more. No less.

Notice the intimacy and constant connectedness that statement implies. You won't see what you're not looking at. You won't hear what you're not listening for. What did Jesus focus upon?

That is the same key for us as well. We will only walk in

power over our sin and our circumstances when we embrace this same kind of intimacy with the Father and say "yes" to Him constantly. Second Corinthians 2:14 tells us that God always leads us in triumph in Christ. But the requirement here is to *be led*.

What does that mean practically? It means practicing obedience. Listen and watch, sense what the Spirit is leading on a moment by moment basis, and obey the leading of the Spirit. First Peter 1:13-15 emphasizes the necessity and the transforming power of simply obeying the Father as faithful children. And once again, the command to be holy means there is a blessing to fulfill that command.

But it all requires relationship, intimate connectedness with the Holy Spirit. Relationship requires effort, yes, but it is not the terribly hard task many believers try to make it. Relationship is life-giving. It changes and adapts and grows, just like any living creature does. Genuine, developing relationships of any kind are less vulnerable to apathetic, heartless choices. There is value involved, and that value leads to a different way of thinking and acting. How much more is this true with the Holy Spirit?

Many believers try to make their own rules in order to stay safe or overcome temptation, but man-made rules are practically worthless compared to the genuine power to be found in intimacy. For example, trying to set and follow a self-made rule against ever eating chocolate basically amounts to a restriction that sooner or later, the flesh will attempt to rebel against and tear down. It has potential to become a source of bitterness.

On the other hand, simply listening to the Lord about whether or not to eat chocolate right now produces more freedom. Instead of "not ever," we may hear "not right now." The Lord is a good Father, and as such, He leads us into what is best, even when we don't understand or necessarily agree. But our eyes remain on Him, just as His remain on us, and the relationship makes submission so much easier than robotically obeying a rule or principle.

Rules vs. Relationship

RULES	RELATIONSHIP
Originate in fear or self-punishment	Originates in love and trust
Attempt to replace the Holy Spirit's leading	Depends on the Holy Spirit for leadership
Are only as strong as your willpower	Brings the power of God to bear
Create a sense of stifling	Promotes the liberty of following the Spirit
Ineffective against the flesh (Gal. 2:23)	Puts the deeds of the flesh to death (Rom. 8:13)

One thing we must never do is violate the God-given laws expressed in His Word. We never have permission to disobey His express command. For example, the Spirit of God will never lead us to steal, since that is a direct violation of the commandment of God. The fact that I know He will forgive me does not justify theft. Willfully breaking God's express commands amounts to rebellion, which as we have already discussed, is equivalent to witchcraft.

Nevertheless, remaining in constant communion with God through His Holy Spirit provides a hedge against such behavior. Through the Holy Spirit's teaching and guidance, we come to better understand the heart of the commandment and the character of our Father. Growing in the understanding of God's character not only produces maturity, but it also magnifies the desire to know even more of Him.

Simply put, nurturing a vibrant and growing relationship with Father, Son, and Holy Spirit empowers us to make different choices. More than that, our obedience as faithful children allows God to reproduce His holiness in our lives on a moment-by-moment basis. That is true freedom.

Righteousness is a Birthright

The Bible teaches us that when we are born again, we are made righteous in God's sight. Jesus is our righteousness (1 Corinthians 1:30), and as such, the source of our righteousness never changes or runs out. However, we also retain a freedom to choose whether or not we will live in that righteousness. Our free will did not cease when we received Jesus as Lord. That is both a blessing, since we can choose to love Him freely, and a liability, since the ability to choose means we can choose wrongly sometimes.

Nevertheless, in terms of our standing with God, as long as we hold to the faith of Jesus as Lord, as the Son of God who died in our place for sin, we are granted through His grace the benefits of righteousness (Colossians 1:19-23). In this sense, righteousness is a "birthright" we receive when we are born again.

With that established, the sad reality is that continuing to participate with sin and bondage amounts to trading in our inheritance of righteousness for something less. Consider the judgment against Esau, found in Hebrews 12:16-17: "lest there be any ***fornicator or profane person*** like Esau, who ***for one morsel of food sold his birthright***. For you know that afterward, when he wanted to inherit the blessing, he was rejected, for he found no place for repentance, though he sought it diligently with tears" (emphasis added).

Esau is judged in this Scripture just like a fornicator or profane person. Something profane is filthy, unworthy, undignified. Why does the Scripture speak so harshly of Esau? Because he traded a blessed birthright for a momentary and passing pleasure. Had he been able to perceive what the Lord intended for Him, he would never have allowed an appetite to cause him to sell his inheritance. His lack of vision combined with his submission to the flesh caused him to forfeit what was rightfully his. The ultimate tragedy, as far as Esau was concerned, was that he didn't even have an opportunity to repent. Thank God for Jesus intervening on our behalf.

Nevertheless, we behave just like Esau when we choose to participate with sin. Our birthright is righteousness with all its benefits and blessings. Yet, we trade that in for a temporary and passing pleasure which never satisfies and only produces death. Looking at it in these terms, it makes absolutely no sense why anyone would ever do such a thing. That's the power and the insidiousness of deception. It makes the temporary look more satisfying than the eternal.

Now that we are aware of that deception, we must realize another tool in our belt that helps us preserve our freedom: we must properly value the inheritance we received from Jesus in the form of righteousness. What benefits and blessings are ours through His sacrifice? Power to live holy; a new identity as a son or daughter, a priest, and a king; the ability to present ourselves to God as an instrument of righteousness; the flavor of Jesus as salt of the earth; the blessing to heal and be healed; the blessing to give what we've been freely given; as well as countless other empowerments and blessings. Wisdom commands us to meditate on what is true, noble, lovely, excellent, or praiseworthy (Philippians 4:8). This godly focus causes the filth to lose its appeal.

While we're on this topic, I would also like to point out that many times what gets us into trouble or opens up the door of temptation is that we participate in thoughts or actions that are not necessarily sinful, but are "borderline." For example, there was a day I thought I'd watch a History Channel special on the Roman emperor, Caligula. As a history enthusiast, I was interested in what the special would say about this literally insane emperor, despite what I knew about him as a sexually perverse person. I felt the check in my spirit saying, "Don't watch this," but I reasoned with myself that the History Channel was not likely to show pornographic material.

In effect, I was watching a show I considered "borderline," since it was not an overtly pornographic program. Nevertheless, the content of the show did stir up ungodly desires. It wasn't that I wanted to see or do any perversions

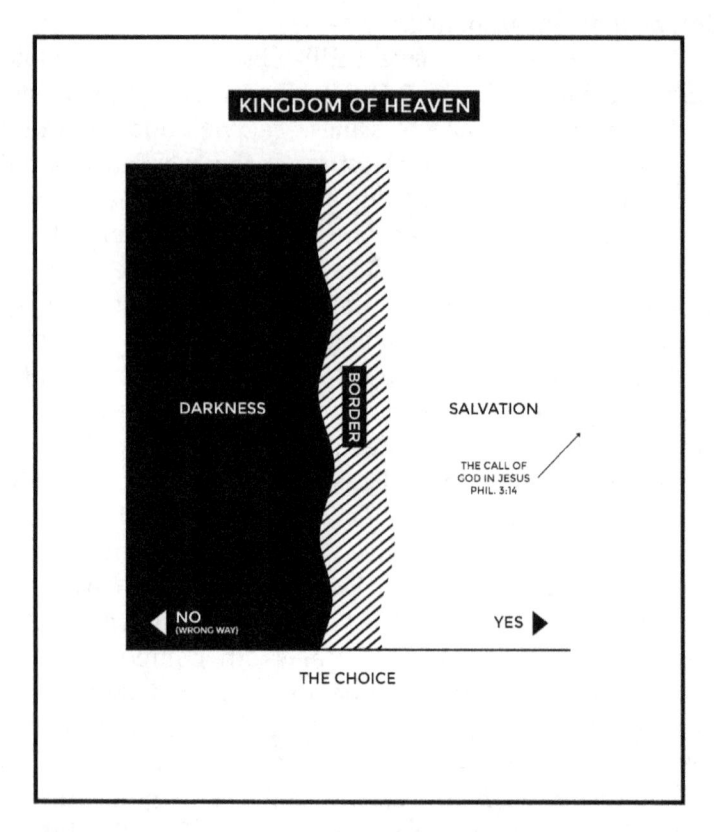

```
┌─────────────────────────────────────┐
│          KINGDOM OF HEAVEN           │
│                                      │
│                    B                 │
│                    O                 │
│   DARKNESS         R    SALVATION    │
│                    D                 │
│                    E    THE CALL OF  │
│                    R    GOD IN JESUS │
│                         PHIL. 3:14 ↗ │
│                                      │
│   ◀ NO                   YES ▶       │
│   (WRONG WAY)                        │
│                                      │
│              THE CHOICE              │
└─────────────────────────────────────┘
```

mentioned in the approximately seven minutes of that show that I watched before I turned it off. It was that I had been disobedient and exposed myself to content that I had no business watching, whether it showed any sexual material or not.

So that kind of activity is what I mean when I say "borderline." The problem with borderline activities is that they focus our attention in the wrong direction. Imagine that you have entered a physical kingdom and you are called to go deeper within that kingdom. If you return to the border or even turn that way, you have turned away from your goal. You've gone the wrong way! It's like that in the Kingdom of Heaven as well. We entered the borders upon salvation, and our call is to go deeper and higher. As we mature, we do go deeper into the Kingdom, which means that if we make the choice to return to the border again, we have made the wrong choice.

That may not sound all that serious, but it really is. In Ezekiel 14:3, God asks the prophet why He should allow people to inquire of Him when they have put things in their paths that they know will cause them to stumble. In other words, to willingly do anything we know could lead to sin is unwise to begin with, but also insulting to the Lord. After all, if He offers blessing and empowerment, but we choose foolishness and filth, He has valid reasons to be angry, especially with those who know better.

> **WEAPONS OF OUR WARFARE:**
>
> *The fear of the Lord. The fear of the Lord is a deep reverence for Who He is. It is an intense honor for the character and the ways of the Lord. Revering King Jesus, the Rider on the white horse from whose mouth the two-edged sword proceeds, will never lead you wrong. Ask the Holy Spirit on a regular basis to release to you a fresh impartation of the fear of the Lord.*

So, once again, the important part of this is to continually choose obedience to God, refusing to trade His gifts for worthless pleasures. Our love for Him and His love for us empower us to make different choices, and if necessary, make changes in our behavior. It may very well mean that we stop watching certain programs or stop going to certain places. I have been led to burn books and destroy DVD's before, even though they were not overtly pornographic.

If there's a rock in your path, you either go around it or move it. Only a foolish person willingly trips over it. If Esau had known what he stood to lose, he would have never eaten that food. We *do* know what is available to us in righteousness, so let's stop trading those blessings for worthless things.

Correction is Good!

One of the biggest enemies of any believer's efforts to stand firm in righteousness is pride. Pride makes confession seem dreadful. It makes us see repentance as either unnecessary or burdensome, and it can even cause us to despise the correction that comes from peers, authorities, and possibly God.

It may well be that not every person struggling with sin and bondage also struggles with pride, but I've experienced it and seen it in enough other people to understand that Satan uses pride to compound the issue when he can. The devil likes to pile on embarrassment and shame, making the believer feel condemned. But that's not how the Holy Spirit works. Holy Spirit brings conviction, which does require a change but also comes with the empowerment and the desire to make that change.

For a believer in Jesus, being corrected is simply a sign that we belong to the family of God. In fact, according to Hebrews 12:5-11, we can all expect to be disciplined by the Lord as He produces His character in us. The Father's ultimate goal is to build us up and produce holiness in our lives.

As the passage points out, discipline and correction are often painful. When I received the discipline of the Lord that summer, as I previously described, I spent about a month feeling completely heartbroken. I did not like it at all, but I could tell that it was producing deep and lasting change in my heart as the Lord also healed me. God knows exactly how to discipline His kids, and He is perfect in this, just as He is in all He does. He can be severe without being harsh. He is firm and unyielding, yet merciful. He breaks what needs to be broken, and heals what needs to be healed.

In order to stay free from the snares of bondage, believers need to learn to embrace the correction and discipline of the Lord. **Oftentimes, this is a trust issue. Do I really trust that God has my best in mind?** Do I believe Him when He says

He is merciful and slow to anger? Will I choose to submit to His ways even when my logical mind is telling me not to?

We must trust Him the way a child trusts a parent. And we must view discipline not as a sign of anger, but as a sign of love and acceptance. The Hebrews 12 passage connects discipline with acceptance. Grant Hill, head worship pastor at The Garden Gathering, has said, "God, Your discipline makes me proud to be Your son." That is the heart of trust. God is making me like Him. Part of that process is His discipline and correction. As He matures me, I get to be proud to carry the family name, so to speak.

And so, the choice becomes the question, will I submit to God in love and trust? Or will I participate with pride and self-righteousness, hiding my sins and refusing His correction?

This issue is not only between the believer and the Lord. It also includes the family of God. Just as discipline issues affect children, parents, and siblings, sin issues affect the body of Christ. As such, we must also view discipline as a family affair among those with whom we are called to walk.

Once again, the goal of discipline within the church is not destruction, but edification. True church leaders following the heart of Jesus will discipline with firmness and love, not according to their own desires, but as led by the Lord. Moreover, since an individual's sin affects those with whom they are in relationship, it only makes sense that those same people get to be a part of the restoration process.

It is wise for a believer to make themselves accountable to those the Lord has placed in his or her life. Your spouse, your fellow believers, and the spiritual authorities in your life are not there by accident. They each have an anointing that God has strategically placed in your life for the purpose of love and mutual edification. As with all decisions we make, it is essential to seek His leading, but opening up with these loved ones and fellow saints can be a powerful part of staying free.

Especially with spouses and spiritual authorities, these believers often have insight into your situation that you have not even been aware of yet. They also have your best interest at heart, along with their genuine love for you. Opening up inside the context of these God-given relationships provides freedom and security. **Think of it like this: if I make myself transparent by willingly living in accountability, I multiply my chances of avoiding the enemy's snares.**

At night, I sometimes walk through my house in the dark before my eyes have adjusted. Navigating that dark haze can be a challenge, even though I'm in familiar territory. I may even make it through to my objective a few times without incident. But sooner or later, despite my best efforts, I bump a picture frame or stub a toe. The simple choice to turn on a light could make this whole adventure so much easier. In like manner, allowing trusted fellow believers to speak into our lives is like turning on the light. Their insight and love can further help me avoid obstacles or traps. As we all know, it is far better to be warned about lurking pieces of furniture rather than bash your shin on them.

The correction of our fellow saints and especially the correction of God make for a formidable defense. However,

> **WEAPONS OF OUR WARFARE:**
>
> *How do you attack while staying protected? One of the best ways is to release God's angels to carry out His Word against the enemy. Psalm 103:20 says they obey the voice of His Word. These mighty and vicious warriors are more than willing to go destroy the emissaries of the enemy before they ever have a chance to get to you. So practically speaking, follow these steps. 1. Speak out and agree with God's Word as led by the Holy Spirit. 2. Dispatch the angels assigned to you to go and carry out God's Word according to His will, in the name of Jesus. 3. Thank God for His mighty hosts who perform His Word.*

in order to fully receive this blessing, we must choose to trust the work of the Lord, especially when He uses those anointed vessels He has placed alongside us to accomplish that work.

Take Heed

History is filled with stories of losers who thought they could not lose. Armies, political candidates, and sports teams can all attest to the necessity of staying humble when things seem to be going well. **Those who believe in their own invincibility often discover that they never had it in the first place.**

In athletics especially, many of the greatest coaches have urged their teams or competitors to stay humble and hungry, even when their teams are performing at peak level. Let's dive into that mentality for a moment.

While coaches may not be right in the middle of the action, they often have a much broader and more thorough view of the competition than the athletes themselves. The coaches recognize weaknesses or bad habits that their trainees may not even believe are present. That's why practices can get so intense: the best coaches spot areas for improvement and drill their athletes until those weak areas become strong. What the coaches realize is that many contests are not decided by skill, but by desire, and sometimes the "better" team loses because the other team's desire to win is stronger. Sometimes the better team on paper gets complacent, and sometimes, the other team just gets lucky. Every coach I've ever known who has coached for a substantial amount of time can tell a horror story about a contest their team lost to an inferior opponent.

That's precisely what happens to us when we step into the sin of pornography. We lose to an inferior opponent who wants us to sin more than we want to remain free. What do we have in common with the great teams who lost to weaker opponents? Once again, it is pride and complacency.

First Corinthians 10:12 offers a simple but urgent warning against thinking too much of ourselves: "Therefore, let him who thinks he stands, take heed lest he fall." In other words, if you think you've got it made, you'd better watch out. Like we've discussed before, one of the biggest mistakes we can make is to let our guard down. No soldier would go into battle without weapons and protective gear. Likewise, no believer walking in freedom can afford to allow pride or complacency to blind us to our weak spots.

So what's the answer to blinding pride and crippling complacency? Humility that keeps us willing to grow and learn, and the fear of the Lord that keeps us dependent upon Him. True humility recognizes that our own strength is inadequate. In the same way that a talented but humble athlete submits to the coach's training, humble believers submit to the teaching and correction of the Holy Spirit. Additionally, the fear of the Lord, that intense reverence for Jesus above all else, makes it especially hard for the enemy to lure us away. If we hate what He hates, we won't do it. If we love what He loves, we won't be as likely to be tempted to act outside His will.

When an enemy army approached the cities of old, the defending soldiers took great care to stay behind the protection of the wall. Walking above the line of the wall made one a target for archers. Similarly, remaining in humility and the fear of the Lord is like the soldier who remains covered by the wall's strong protection. Pride tempts us to stand tall, which gives the enemy opportunity to shoot us down.

At this point, someone is probably thinking, "Now hold on a minute! Didn't you say we had to believe we could be completely free? And now you're saying we have to watch out and stay protected. Which is it?"

Just as it is a huge error to go on believing that we can never break free from sexual sin, it is just as grievous a mistake to believe that we can never fall into it again. Jesus's analogy of the narrow road applies here. On one side of the narrow road are those poor souls who won't come up out of the sludge because they do not believe it is possible. On the other side are those prideful people who crashed because they thought they had it made. True freedom is found in steadfastly remaining on the narrow road.

We truly are in a superior position that Jesus has given to us. We have a strong fortress of defense. We get to walk in the glorious freedom of the children of God. In Jesus, we can be and indeed are victorious over sin. And yet, despite all of these wonderful truths, we can still choose to participate with the works of darkness.

Remember the lesson taught by the great sports teams who lost. Complacency and belief in one's superiority are two of the main ingredients in the recipe for defeat. Victorious and invincible are not synonyms. We may not always have to fight, but we must always remain vigilant. Therefore, let us take heed.

Get Vicious

Everything we've discussed so far might very well be classified as defensive maneuvers in the battle against bondage. Now I'd like to shift the focus to the offensive side.

There's a sports saying that goes something like this: "The best defense is a good offense." While I find that statement debatable even in the sports arena, there is truth to the idea that one of the best ways to defend territory is to attack the attackers *before* they arrive. Returning to the analogy of ancient warfare, if soldiers were tasked with defending a city wall, it would be in their best interest to attack the sieging army well before it got to the city. The enemy can't launch the bombardment if they never get in range.

In the spiritual sense, it is much the same way. Rather than simply responding to attacks that have already come, the believer would be wise to cut off those attacks before they arrive. Ephesians 6 describes some of the armor and weaponry available to every believer in Jesus. However, many of us only put these weapons to use in the moment they're needed.

The better strategy is to keep these weapons polished and sharp and in constant use. For example, if we constantly allow the helmet of God's salvation to guard our minds, we are less susceptible to attack. Practically speaking, we can choose to agree with the fullness of what salvation means: through the grace of God and the sacrifice of Jesus, we are forgiven, cleansed, made whole, set free, and blessed to fulfill our purpose as God's adopted children. Our unrelenting focus on these truths is like a helmet that protects our minds from the lies of the devil.

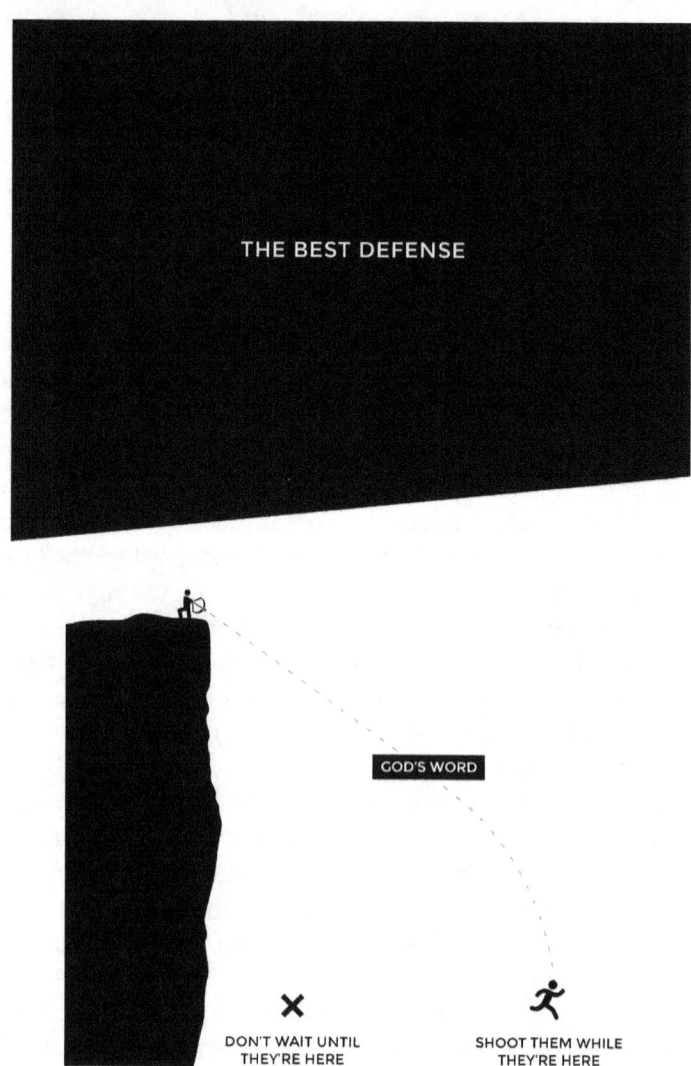

THE BEST DEFENSE

GOD'S WORD

✗ DON'T WAIT UNTIL THEY'RE HERE

🏃 SHOOT THEM WHILE THEY'RE HERE

Similarly, if we constantly use the sword of the Spirit, God's Word, by reading it, believing it, and speaking it over ourselves and our lives, our swords stay sharp and the Word has its effect (it never returns void). When we fully agree with God's Word and release it with our mouths, it's like a shower of arrows we send out into the enemy's ranks. With the Holy Spirit guiding our shots, we mow down the other army before it ever has the chance to attack. These are just two examples of the weapons God has made available to those who believe.

Furthermore, our willingness and ability to use these weapons make the enemy much less eager to target us. Remember how Satan doesn't like to attack strength? It only makes sense then to keep ourselves strong in the Lord and in the power of His might. That's one form of offense that bears much fruit.

Another form of offense is not to merely chase off those scouts and chiselers that like to test our walls, but to utterly destroy them. As we've previously noted, 2 Corinthians 10:4-5 says our weapons are mighty to pull down strongholds, cast down arguments and high things that exalt themselves against the knowledge of God, and bring every thought into captivity to the obedience of Jesus. That's powerful. That means I can go disassemble those siege machines while they're out there in the field. I can cast down lies or lying spirits that want to keep me from knowing God better. And I can even take thoughts captive, making them prisoner to Jesus. Imagine what He will do to those things that attack His beloved! (Seriously, take a minute to imagine.)

The encouragement here is to engage in this battle not simply as a defender, but as an attacker as well. We want to have strong walls, and we want our arrows flying out at the enemy too. We want him to stay off in the distance where he can't reach us.

The Lord has also encouraged me lately to speak His Word concerning what He likes to do to His enemies. Psalm 3:5-8 describes the Lord breaking the teeth of the wicked. Psalm 37:17 says the arms of the wicked shall be broken. Psalm

10:15 affirms the arms of the wicked being broken as the Lord pursues them until they are destroyed.

In addition, according to Psalm 103:20-21, we also have an army of angels waiting eagerly to carry out the Word of the Lord. It can be extremely encouraging to imagine a mighty angel of Heaven spending its fury against one of the pitiful minions of hell just because that little minion had the audacity to mess with you, one of King Jesus's favorites.

Practically speaking, I encourage you to put God's battle words into your mouth as you pray. For example, if you find an ungodly thought flitting through your mind, don't let it get away with a warning! Try this instead: "Father, in the name of Jesus I bind that thought and destroy its power over me. I plead the blood of Jesus to cleanse my mind entirely from its effect. I command that thought to be captured and taken prisoner in Jesus name. Let the evil source of that thought be captured and bound as well, and may its arms and teeth be broken. I command the angels assigned to me to carry out these words and to take that evil spirit where Jesus commands it to go, never to return or minister to me in any way from this moment forth, in Jesus's name!"

That's not the only way to go about it, but just try it out and see if your spirit does not rise up within you like a warrior. When you pray this way, you're not being arrogant. You're taking what God has already said and releasing it like a missile. The enemy hates this because it shows how weak he truly is against the might of the LORD GOD.

I recommend copying the prayer above onto a note card or writing it as a note in your smart phone. Keep it close at hand so that you can at least have a model for those moments in your day when vicious warfare may become a necessity. I also urge you to ask the Holy Spirit to add to this prayer or to give you your own way of praying over yourself. It is wise to have a vast arsenal of weapons at your disposal.

When we not only defend our walls vigilantly but also are willing to use the offensive weapons God has placed at our disposal, we're sending the message to the hordes of hell, "If you attack me or what is mine, it will not go well for you. I will not tolerate assassins in my house. Neither will I tolerate any spirit that tries to destroy me or what is mine!" As a benchmark for how vicious you ought to be against the spiritual enemies that come to tempt you, consider how you'd react if it were a human being. How would you deal with a man who stood on your doorstep, tried to get you to do things you hated, threatened your home, ministry, and marriage, and made your spouse feel like trash? Now take that and multiply by ten and you've got a good start.

It is important to remember, though, that we win the war by the leading of the Holy Spirit. I do not recommend that you go out looking to pick a fight. You might pick one the Lord did not send you into, and that will not go well. We always stay within the strong fortress of God's will.

Nevertheless, when the enemy trespasses on your territory, it would behoove you to rise up, get vicious, and take the fight to him.

Jesus Defeated Temptation, Too

It is common knowledge that Jesus triumphed over sin and death. What fewer people realize is that Jesus defeated temptation as well.

After His baptism in water, Jesus was led into the wilderness to be tempted. Satan tried to tempt Jesus to prove Who He was by asking Him to do tricks. The father of lies attempted to persuade Jesus to test God's Word. The accuser offered Jesus the world if He would just worship the devil rather than God. It's hard to imagine what else the devil may have tried on our Lord. After all, Hebrews 5:15 tells us that Jesus was tempted in every way just as we are, but did not sin. In other words, Satan lost.

That's one reason our faithful High Priest is so willing to help us in time of need. When we approach Him with how the enemy is attacking us, Jesus can say every time, "I was tempted that way also. Now receive My grace and My help to overcome!"

But as you well know, the temptation in the wilderness

was not the end of the story. Jesus still had more overcoming to do, found in Matthew 26:36-46. This was Gethsemane, the place of the greatest temptation Jesus ever faced. At Gethsemane, Jesus was face to face with the reality that He was about to be betrayed, handed over, tortured beyond recognition, and ultimately killed. More than that, He was about to have to take all the sins of the world for all generations onto Himself.

Imagine for a moment the heartfelt prayer of Jesus in that moment: "God if there is ANY WAY, please let this pass from me." The description of the event says Jesus's sweat became like drops of blood. This was the devil's best shot. None of us will ever face this level of temptation. And Jesus still won.

When Jesus surrendered to the Father's will, saying, "Not my will but Yours be done," He overcame the greatest temptation the world has ever known. Then He went to the cross to shed His blood to end that war once and for all.

You see, Jesus shedding His blood paid for not only the consequence of sin, but it also destroyed the power of the temptations that draw us toward sin. Hebrews 12:3-4 says, "For consider Him who endured such hostility from sinners against Himself, lest you become weary and discouraged in your souls. You have not yet resisted to bloodshed, striving against sin." Jesus endured hostility on our behalf. None of us has shed our blood striving against sin, but Jesus has. **Through the blood of Jesus, we are covered by the very thing that purchased our righteousness, which means that temptation and sin have no power to dominate us whatsoever.**

That's powerful! That truth flies in the face of the notion that we as believers have to live with temptation as if it were a given. Jesus defeated temptation even before He defeated sin. If we can live lives free from sin, then we can overcome the power of temptation through Jesus's blood as well.

Now, I'm not teaching you that temptation won't still try to come. What I am teaching is that we don't have to succumb to it. Moreover, we as believers don't even have to put up with temptation. We have weapons; let's use them!

Practically speaking, we use our weapons to destroy the power of temptation, then by faith we fill ourselves up with the blessings God has promised. For example, if I'm being tempted to watch a show I know I shouldn't watch, I can pray to destroy the power of that temptation by the blood of Jesus, then ask to be filled with peace and satisfaction by the grace of God.

An important concept to keep in the forefront of our minds is that God's power to keep us is greater than the power of Satan to tempt us. In John 14:15-18, Jesus describes the Helper He sent to us upon His return to Heaven. This is the Holy Spirit, the very power by which God created the heavens and the earth, and these verses teach that He will live inside us. Compared to the Holy Spirit, Satan's got nothing. **Our Helper, who abides with us, is infinitely greater than the tempter. You mess with me, you get Him.**

Moreover, Romans 8:26-27 describes how the Spirit helps us in our weaknesses and makes constant intercession for us. He never tires, and He never gives up. He has a permanent audience with our Father and Defender. This should be a major encouragement. My Helper prays for me, and Jesus listens! I am set up to win.

But why do so many believers still struggle so much with temptation? Part of it is that repentance needs to come. We must continually allow the Word of God to transform our minds so that our agreement is no longer with temptation or the enemy, but with the promises of our Father. Too many believers have simply agreed that temptation and sin are necessary parts of our lives. Jesus says otherwise.

The Bible says clearly that Jesus came to destroy the work of the devil (1 John 3:8). He accomplished His mission in full. If temptation is the work of the devil, which it certainly is, then Jesus has destroyed its power. Therefore, walking in freedom and abiding with the Holy Spirit really still comes back to the simple but profound question: to whom will I choose to submit?

It's time to believe what God's Word says and come out of those agreements with the power of temptation. Get vicious about it. Resist the devil and he will flee.

But What If I Stumble?

This is a question a lot of people have when they come out of bondage. They remember the intense draw those sins had on them, and it's hard not to wonder if it will ever happen again. So what's the guarantee that it won't?

We've already talked about the proper mentality – rejecting the notion that you will always struggle with sin while remaining humble and vigilant. That by itself will go a long way towards ensuring you don't step back into that old bondage.

Another important part is to cultivate the character of Jesus along with the fear of the Lord. Speak aloud that you love the things Jesus loves and hate the things Jesus hates. Allow the Word to transform your thoughts and desires so that they match His. And let the fear of the Lord have its way any time you're considering walking those shady paths toward temptation. Ask Holy Spirit to reveal how Jesus feels about it, and He will show you.

Your worst enemies, as we have noted, are pride and apathy. Walking closely with people you trust can help you avoid these traps. Invite those you trust most to speak into your life and correct you when they sense pride rising up or when they can tell you're not holding up your weapons. It may hurt in the moment to be told you're getting complacent or acting pridefully, but if that causes you to examine yourself and rise up, it has done its work. Proverbs 27:6 says, "Faithful are the wounds of a friend, but the kisses of an enemy are deceitful." I'd rather my friend wound me than have an enemy kiss me. Remember, transparency gives the enemy nowhere to hide and further protects you from sin.

"Yeah, but what if it *does* happen again? What then?"

In the event that you do stumble in sin again, it is not the end of the world. Is it serious? Absolutely. Remember that we cannot afford to write off willful sin as a small thing. Nevertheless, Jesus is in the business of redemption and there is no sin He is not willing to forgive (other than blasphemy of the Holy Spirit). So here are some practical questions and steps to take in the event that you stumble:

1. Have you confessed to God and received forgiveness?
If not, do it and trust in His mercy.
2. Have you forgiven and released yourself?
Be sure not to hold grudges against yourself. That's doing the enemy's work for him.
3. If you're married, have you opened up with your spouse about it?
You cannot hide this without consequences.
4. Have you contacted those in authority and/or close relationship with you?
They can be very powerful in prayer and in making sure condemnation does not spring up.
5. Have you sought the counsel of the Holy Spirit?
Think back to any place you know you walked in disobedience. Confess, repent, and ask forgiveness as needed.
6. Are there strongholds and/or spirits at work?
Ask Holy Spirit to show you any stronghold you may have rebuilt. Ask Holy Spirit to reveal any spirit at work through those strongholds. Confess and repent. Renounce all participation with strongholds and spirits. Ask for the cleansing of Jesus. Then destroy those strongholds and cast out those spirits in Jesus' name.
7. Is there any area the Lord is asking you to add/change/remove?
Ask the Lord for His counsel and obey what He shows you. This may also involve church discipline or personal discipline from Jesus. It's not punishment, but it will bring about fruit if you submit to it.

8. Are you continuing to hold on to and believe for your freedom?
If you have given up on it in any way, repent immediately. The cross was not deficient in anything. Your freedom has been purchased, and you get to live in it. Receive this truth as often as needed.

Always and everywhere, give God the glory He deserves. He loves you. He wants great things for you. He chose you specifically. You are the apple of His eye. He gave His Son not just to hide your sin, but to destroy and remove it. The blood of Jesus has gained you access to God's throne. The Holy Spirit empowers you for freedom and victory. You are beloved! Worship God and thank Him for all these truths. Allow His Spirit and His great mercy to wash you entirely.

And never stop loving Him.

Only Love Can Win

If you have read this far, then I bless you in your commitment to walking in freedom. I know this journey has not been a pleasant one, since it surely has not been pleasant for me, but I am convinced that my God is able and willing to redeem to the uttermost all the time we have given to other lovers and work even that for our good. I'm looking forward to what He has in store for us in the future, and I only look back for the purpose of sharing my testimony and empowering others to walk free. I look back to see where God was. I look forward to see where He's leading me. In the moment, I trust that He is with me always. He was, He is, He is to come.

For the longest time, I failed to truly understand what it meant to be loved by the Father. True, from the moment I was first saved until this very day, Holy Spirit has been working on and in me to reveal the Father's love. That's His job, after all. But I still had a mindset of performance, works-based faith, the notion that I somehow had to earn what He was giving me. That proved a major stumbling block on my road to freedom from bondage.

Since I had not received God's love fully as a matter of simple faith, I still tried to insert myself in the equation. I felt that I had something to add that was lacking. From this side of things, that seems really silly. I won't list all the methods I tried in order to break free, but suffice it to say, I have learned that no form of motivation, no amount of effort, is sufficient to overcome bondage. It wasn't until I truly began to lay hold of the Father's love that freedom began to reign in my life.

That was actually the number one thing Jesus modeled as well. He showed what life could look like if a child of God made loving God and being loved by Him the number one priority at all times. What a testimony He gave to the Father's perfect love.

In John 14, Jesus is preparing Himself and His disciples for His upcoming torture and death. In this chapter and the chapters that follow, He teaches them of the Holy Spirit, urges them to abide in Him, pleads for them to allow His Word to abide in their hearts, tells them plainly what will soon occur, and prays for them mightily. I find it encouraging that, even though He knew what He was about to endure, Jesus still loved His disciples enough to prepare them. More than that, He loved the Father enough to focus on bringing Him glory.

In John 14:30-31, Jesus tells the disciples, "I will no longer talk much with you, for the ruler of this world is coming, and he has nothing in Me. But that the world may know that I love the Father, and as the Father gave Me commandment, so I do." There are two parts of this I want to highlight.

First, Jesus notes that Satan is coming, but the devil has nothing in Him. What a statement to make. **There was not a single area the devil could influence in Jesus's mind, body, or heart.** He had nothing! Jesus had given His Father every part of Himself, so Satan had not one iota of opportunity in Jesus's life. My friends, that should be our ultimate goal as well. Complete surrender to the love of the Father allows Him to produce His perfect character in us. Yes it is a process, but our willingness to follow the model of Jesus in surrender can accelerate that process. Jesus said we could do what He did, so may I suggest that abiding with Holy Spirit, abiding in God's love to the point where the devil just gives up is part of what we're called to pursue? At any rate, Jesus loved the Father to the point where He could truly say, "Satan has nothing in me." I want that for myself, too.

Secondly, Jesus reveals His greatest motivation for going to the cross: "But that the *world may know that I love the Father*, and as the Father gave me commandment, so I do." While it is true that Jesus went to the cross because of His great love for the world, that was actually secondary to His greater purpose. In this moment of preparation, Jesus testified that He would obey God's command and go to the cross to proclaim to the world that He loved His Father. He further urged the disciples to submit to the Holy Spirit because the Holy Spirit would show them how to love. In His prayer, He passionately asked the Father to glorify Himself. At Gethsemane, Jesus prayed in complete submission, "Not my will, but Yours be done." Simply put, Jesus overcame every temptation of the enemy by love. He knew He was loved by God, and He loved God with all His heart, all His mind, all His soul, and all His strength.

Hebrews 5:7-8 describes how Jesus, "when He had offered up prayers and supplications, with vehement cries and tears to Him who was able to save Him from death, and was heard because of His godly fear, though He was a Son, yet He learned obedience by the things which He suffered." In other words, Jesus loved the Father so much He obeyed to the point of death.

When you have a heart like that, nothing can touch you.

If we follow the example Jesus set, we come to know that love is the only motivator that truly works. Other motivators, worthwhile though they may be, do not carry the same power that love carries to truly and permanently transform our minds, hearts, and even our bodies. Inspiration slowly fades. Fear is not helpful because it paralyzes in the moment and dissipates over time so that it does not produce godly fruit. Anger fails to produce God's righteousness. Grief makes us weak and heavy. Even godly sorrow is meant to produce the fruits of repentance, one of which is love.

Love is the only motivator that never fails. That is at least a part of why Jesus commanded us to abide in love (John 15:9). Love for Jesus overshadows and eliminates affection for past lovers. Love endures where other motivators can't. Love empowers us to obey the Father, and obeying the Father produces more love.

In addition to this powerful cycle of loving and being loved by the Father, our love for others is also a powerful weapon. We love our spouses, our fellow believers, our churches, and even ourselves with the kind of love Jesus produces as we love Him.

In summation, the only way to get free and to know that you are truly free from bondage and sin is to fully engage in a lifestyle of love. That's how Jesus did it, and that's how we can do it too.

Practically speaking, living a lifestyle of love means sacrificing the pleasure of the flesh on a moment by moment basis. Can I get real? I really, really, really like ice cream. But there are times when I feel the Holy Spirit saying "no" to ice cream. Is ice cream sinful? I don't think so. Nevertheless, He has good reason if He's saying that I shouldn't have it. I may not necessarily agree, and I may have good logical reasons why I'm free to eat ice cream. But out of love for Him, I choose to submit.

The point is, I love Him, so I obey. That brings with it blessing and peace. And it doesn't create a rule against ice cream. It is relationship, not dead religion.

In the same manner, focusing on the genuine love you have for Jesus, for your friends, for your spouse, empowers you to choose differently than you have in the past. I don't want my wife feeling insecure, so I proactively ask her to shut off the internet app on my phone any time she travels. It's not that I'm afraid that I'll stumble, but more that I don't want the enemy to have an opportunity to attack either of us. I do not tolerate sinful desires because not only do I not want them affecting me, I don't want those assassins to have access to my beloved family in Christ.

Do you get the idea? I love God so I can submit with joy. I love my wife so I let that empower me to choose better. I love my church family, so I am motivated to protect them. On and on it goes.

Love, my friends, is your greatest weapon. Love the Lord with all your heart, all your soul, all your mind, and all your strength, and love your neighbor as yourself. Don't forget to love yourself, too. We all matter. When you can do these things, to whatever extent you are able, then you will know you are walking in freedom.

By now, I hope you are convinced that freedom really is a possibility. It is for freedom that Christ has made us free (Galatians 5:1). We have been blessed to overcome deception and temptation, empowered to destroy the works of our enemy, and loved with a love beyond our comprehension.

Our Father loves us, and He wants us to win.

May you break free from the cycles you've lived in and escape to a wide place with the Lord. May your mind and heart be cleansed and healed by the love of our Father. May your eyes be opened to recognize deception and may your spirit rise up as a mighty warrior within you. May you truly see the deliverance of the Lord manifest in your life. And may you stand fast in the liberty by which Christ has made you free.

"Now to Him who is able to keep you from stumbling, and to present you faultless before the presence of His glory with exceeding joy, to God our Savior, Who alone is wise, be glory and majesty, dominion and power, both now and forever. Amen" (Jude 24-25).

He is able if we are willing. Godspeed.

Appendix 1: The Gospel: Step One to Freedom

While there are many organizations and individuals in the secular world working to free people from the snare of pornography, all with varying degrees of success, the ultimate key to true freedom from this sinister form of bondage is faith in the Lord Jesus. I respect the efforts those people are making, but the reality is that pornography is a physical manifestation of a spiritual battle, and the only way to win a spirit-battle is through the spirit. Jesus is Lord of the spiritual realm (Colossians 1:16; 2:9-10). Therefore, He is the only means by which anyone can hope to be saved from the grip of pornography or any form of bondage.

This brief chapter is not intended to be an in-depth teaching on the fullness of the Gospel. That would require an entire book to itself. Instead, this chapter outlines the Biblical truths that lead us to salvation and Kingdom empowerment. If you have not received Jesus as Lord, these Scriptures show you how and why you must do so. If you have already received Jesus as Lord, enjoy being reminded of the foundation for your faith.

The best way to approach this chapter is to pick up a Bible and go look up each Scripture reference for yourself. Allow God's Word to speak to your heart, and ask the Holy Spirit to reveal the deep meaning in each passage and verse.

In the beginning, God made Adam and Eve and blessed them to have dominion over the earth (Genesis 1:26-28).

When Adam sinned, he surrendered his dominion to Satan, and sin entered the world (Genesis 3; Romans 5:12-17; Luke 4:5-7).

God already had a plan for the redemption of mankind

from Satan's power (Genesis 3:14-15 - The Seed prophesied points to Jesus, who would crush Satan's head).

God gave the Law as a way to separate His chosen people from the world and to bless them. The Law is also a tutor that pointed out our need for Christ by demonstrating that no man can live righteously by himself (Deuteronomy 5:1-22; Deuteronomy 6:17-19; Romans 6:7; Galatians 3:19-25).

The prophets began to speak of a coming Messiah who would free people from sin and bring them back to the Father (Isaiah 53; Jeremiah 23:5-7; Psalm 22).

It is clear that every person has sinned and that the just reward of sin is spiritual death – separation from the Presence of God and ultimately, eternity in hell (Romans 3:21-23; Romans 6:23; Ephesians 2:1-3; Colossians 1:21).

At the right time, Jesus came to take away the sins of the world and reconcile mankind to God (John 1:29: John 3:16-17; Colossians 1:22-23; Romans 5:8-9).

We are saved from death and hell by faith in Jesus (Romans 10:8-9; 1 Peter 2:24; Ephesians 2:4-9).

Salvation also means we are delivered from our enemies, set free from oppression, healed, and made whole in every way (Isaiah 53; 2 Corinthians 5:17-21; Luke 8:40-48; Acts 10:38; John 14:27).

Jesus regained all authority lost by Adam and commissioned His followers to go out into the world sharing the good news (Matthew 28:18-20; Mark 16:15-16).

The Holy Spirit continually guides believers to live as Jesus did (John 14:26; Romans 8:1-17; 1 Corinthians 2:12-16; 2 Corinthians 2:14; 2 Corinthians 3: 5-6; Galatians 5:22-25).

The Holy Spirit gives gifts to empower believers to share the gospel and to encourage and build the body of Christ (1 Corinthians 12, 13, and 14; Ephesians 4:11-16; Romans 12:6-8).

The body of Christ is to advance the Kingdom of Heaven until Jesus comes to reign (Psalm 145:13; Isaiah 9:6-7; Matthew 6:9-10; Hebrews 12:18-29).

Jesus also promised to baptize His followers in the Holy Spirit so that we would receive power to continue His ministry (Matthew 3:11; John 14:12; 16-17; John 16:5-15; Luke 24:49; Acts 1:4-8).

If you read these Scriptures from start to finish, you begin to see the full picture of the Good News. Mankind sinned, which separated us from God and invited sin into the world. Satan stole the authority intended for mankind. God's plan for redemption was already in place. He gave the law to show that people cannot live righteously apart from His help. The prophets further testified of the coming King who would save His people.

Then, Jesus was made manifest to the world so that all who believe in Him would receive eternal life and be reconciled to God. Furthermore, He took back the authority Adam had surrendered to Satan, then commissioned His followers to preach His gospel to the whole world. To help us accomplish that mission, Jesus gave us the Holy Spirit as a Helper to empower us to walk in freedom, bear witness to the glory of Jesus, and lead others to salvation through faith in Christ. The Holy Spirit also gives gifts so that the body of Christ can encourage and edify one another while we wait for the return of our glorious King.

So what must one do to be saved? First, we must admit to ourselves and confess before God that we have sinned and are therefore worthy of condemnation. We must agree with His Word that there is not one person who is righteous by our own efforts, and that only Jesus lived sinless and perfect. We must acknowledge that we need someone to save us since we cannot save ourselves. We must ask for and receive His forgiveness.

Second, we must believe in our hearts that Jesus is who He says He is – the Son of God who died in our place to remove our sins. He is the Lord of all the earth, worthy of our surrender. He is the One who loves us enough to bring us home to the Father, though He had to pay for it with His own blood.

Next, we must confess with our mouths while agreeing in our hearts that Jesus is Lord. This confession involves surrendering our lives to Him as master. We die to ourselves, meaning our old way of living has passed away, and we now choose daily to allow Him to live in us and through us. We submit to His Word, His guidance, and His Holy Spirit.

Finally, we ask Him to fill us with His Holy Spirit. By faith we trust that He has done what we have asked Him to do, and we begin to live for His glory.

If you want to receive Jesus as Lord, you can pray something like this:

Father, in the name of Jesus, I confess to You that I have sinned against You. I have done wrong in Your sight and I am fully deserving of death. But God, I believe that Jesus is Your Son, who came to Earth, lived a sinless life, died upon the cross in my place and for my sins, and that You resurrected Him from the dead. I believe His sacrifice paid the price for my sins so that I could come home to You. So Lord, because of what Jesus did for me, I ask You to forgive me for all my sins, and I receive Your forgiveness now by faith. I confess from my heart that Jesus Christ is Lord, and I surrender my life fully to Him. Lord Jesus, my life belongs to You. I invite You to make Your home in me and to live in and through me. I ask You to remove anything that does not belong in me. I choose to submit to Your Lordship in all areas of my life. I ask You now Lord to fill me with Your Holy Spirit. Thank You for forgiving me. Thank You for saving me. Thank You for living in and through me. I love You Lord, and I am grateful that You love me enough to receive me to Yourself. I pray these things in the name of Jesus Christ, my Lord. Amen.

There are no magic words and there is no "right" way to pray, but if you prayed in this manner, believing what you prayed in your heart, you have been born again to a new life in Jesus. I encourage you to tell anyone you know who has been praying for you what you have done. It is also essential that you get connected to a Bible-believing congregation so that you can continue to learn and grow alongside other believers in Christ.

Once you have been born again, the next step is to receive the baptism of the Holy Spirit. I recommend talking to Spirit-filled believers about it and getting them to pray for you. I also recommend that you begin immediately to pray for God's guidance and for understanding of this important matter. However, you can ask Jesus to baptize you in His Spirit right where you are. If you ask, you will receive.

For further study on the Gospel of the Kingdom, the baptism of the Holy Spirit, and other essentials for believers in Christ visit the Garden's "Teachings" page at this web address: http://thegardenstc.org/contentpage.php?id=8&itemId=3#Who Am I in Christ.

LIBERATED

Appendix 2: Deliverance Ministry: We Do Not Struggle Against Flesh and Blood

As with the appendix summarizing the Gospel, this chapter is not intended to be a full, in-depth teaching on deliverance. There are many excellent books already out there that powerfully instruct believers in how to rid their lives from the influence of the enemy. Dr. Nancy Hadley's *It's Only a Shadow* provides straightforward testimony about the reality of spiritual warfare and is very useful for those seeking to learn about the spirit realm. Dr. Henry Malone's *Shadow Boxing* is a game-changing reference for those believers who want to learn the practical ins and outs of ministering deliverance. These books and books like them will help anyone interested in diving in deeper to the nature and methods of deliverance.

In this brief summary, I'll do my best to concisely answer some common questions concerning the ministry of deliverance and why it is such a vital tool for any believer who genuinely wants to walk like Jesus.

What is Deliverance?

At a basic level, deliverance involves three basic parts:
1. The believer identifies areas where he has surrendered power, agreement, or influence to the enemy. In addition, the believer identifies where the enemy has intruded.
2. The believer identifies the root causes of that surrendered power, etc. Through repentance, forgiveness, and healing, the believer pulls up those roots (or tears down the stronghold).

3. The believer, now healed, forgiven, and choosing repentance, casts out whatever enemies were operating in their lives.

Often, believers will go through a "deliverance session." This means a time set aside for the express purpose of receiving deliverance as outlined above. There will almost always be one or two fellow believers who support and minister to the one receiving deliverance ministry. Deliverance sessions may take place in homes, churches, or anywhere the group is not likely to be interrupted or distracted. It is important that the environment be peaceful and conducive to prayer and listening to the guidance of the Holy Spirit.

Prior to going through a deliverance session, and even during the session, a person may spend a great deal of time searching his or her heart and allowing the Holy Spirit to highlight fruit being produced that is not of Him. While the deliverance session is taking place, there is an ongoing conversation between those ministering and the one being ministered to wherein all are actively listening to the Holy Spirit for direction. Sometimes, the one receiving ministry talks a bit, then receives ministry in the form of tearing down strongholds and casting out demons. There may be time for the person to both forgive others and receive forgiveness for sin. Sometimes, the one receiving ministry opens up for a long period of time, followed by a long period of ministry. The model and method vary each time, but the purpose is the same: seek the enemy and his hiding place, and through the direction and power of the Holy Spirit, destroy the place and remove the "thing."

What do you mean when you say someone is "demonized?"

Being demonized, or having demons, is a way of expressing that demonic spirits can influence and affect someone's life without fully possessing them. Many believers and non-believers are demonized, rather than being demon-possessed. In this case, the demon has obtained a dwelling place in the person's mind, will, emotions, or physical body. The demon influences and affects that dwelling place, working to create evil fruit, such as ungodly thoughts or actions. If the demon is not removed, the fruit it produces can become a stronghold, meaning a sinful pattern of thinking or acting that is impossible to destroy by willpower alone.

I've been taught that Christians can't have demons. Is this true?

Simply put, no. The belief that a Christian is exempt from having demons is responsible for a great many sincere, born-again, Bible-believing saints remaining stuck in cycles of sin which they absolutely despise. These believers are doing the equivalent of tearing down a house but not making the occupants leave. If the occupants are determined to stay, they'll just rebuild the house and go on doing whatever they were doing. This is why some believers walk free from sin patterns for a time, but then, seemingly inexplicably, find themselves drawn to the very sin they have tried so hard to escape.

There's another analogy I find useful for describing this situation as well. Imagine a believer with a rope tied around his waist. On the other end of the rope is another person holding the rope fast. The rope represents a sinful behavior, and the one holding the rope represents a demon. No matter how fast the believer runs, they're still tied with the rope and they'll end up going in circles. The strong-willed believers may even be able to drag that demon in the direction they feel called to go, but eventually fatigue sets in and the demon does its best to drag them back in the direction they came. This is the back-and-forth a lot of believers struggle with in their walk.

Now, a believer has some choices here. He can cut the rope, which is his choice to repent from the sin. That's a good thing to do by the way. That will purchase some freedom, at least for a time. But that demon won't just give up and go away because the believer repented. He'll chase the guy until he can get that rope back in place again, and then the old situation is right back where it was before. The believer gained some ground, walked in some freedom, and then found themselves in the same sin. Often, this turns into major condemnation, shame, and guilt for those in this situation.

On the other hand, a believer can kill the one holding the rope. Again, this is a good thing to do. This gives the believer the opportunity to make forward progress without the extra weight of that demon slowing them down. But the guy still has a rope trailing behind him. Those sinful desires, thought patterns, and behaviors didn't go away just because he took the demon out. All it takes is some other demon to come along and pick up that rope, and the man is right back where he was.

Using this analogy, the best course of action is to cast the demon out and destroy the rope. Repentance and casting out demons give the believer the opportunity to make forward progress without the past hindrances. Of course, the believer can choose to pick up another rope, or invite another demon to chase him, but those who truly leave the rope and the demon behind can walk in true freedom without the fear of going back.

Is there Biblical evidence to support deliverance?

Tons of it. It would take a whole book to really thoroughly explore. But let me point to some things for you to consider.

Ephesians 6:12 makes it clear that "we do not struggle against flesh and blood, but against principalities, against powers, against the rulers of the darkness of this age, against spiritual hosts of wickedness in the heavenly places." In other words, if we're sinning, it's not only because we're terrible sinners. We're up against an army of darkness, complete with pesky minions and former glorious angels now turned servants of Satan. That's a hard reality, but it's reality.

Now what do you think those spirits are trying to

accomplish? They're following the job description of their master: steal, kill, destroy. These spirits will use whatever means necessary. They know no quarter or mercy. They will lie, cheat, tempt, deceive, and do whatever it takes to keep believers from advancing the Kingdom of Heaven. The armor of God described in Ephesians 6 is not an option if you want to walk victoriously – it is essential.

Another passage that points to the need for deliverance is 2 Corinthians 10:4-5. This book makes reference to this passage several times, but for now, let's focus on the parts that show why deliverance is necessary.

Verse four describes the pulling down of strongholds. A basic definition for a stronghold is a sinful pattern of thought or behavior. Our sinful thoughts and actions are the building material the enemy uses to build his house, his place of operation, in our souls or bodies. This is the first reason deliverance is so necessary: it helps the believer identify and destroy the enemy's base of operation.

Verse five builds on that thought by pointing out the need to cast down "arguments and every high thing that exalts itself against the knowledge of God." Arguments are easily understood as those lies the enemy tries to get us to believe about God or about ourselves. The verse makes clear that the objective of this tool is to cause believers not to truly know who God is. Deliverance is one way believers cast the lies of the enemy down so that those lies no longer affect how the believer lives.

The other part of the verse refers to a "high thing that exalts itself." If it's really a thing/object, how does it exalt itself? It is apparent that these high things we're to be casting down are actually beings, and if they're exalting themselves against the knowledge of God, it's not hard to decipher what kind of being we're talking about.

Continuing on this line of thought, it's not hard to see why the Lord included discerning of spirits among the inventory of spiritual gifts. In 1 Corinthians 12:4-11, Paul describes many of the ways the Holy Spirit works in the body of believers. Verse ten says, "to another the working of miracles, to another prophecy, to another discerning of spirits..." There are two points I'd like to make about this. First, in verse seven, the passage says these gifts are given for the profit of all. In other words, the ability to discern spirits is meant to benefit both non-believers and the church. This becomes especially clear when considering the second thing I'd like to point out: the passage, just like the book of Ephesians and the entire book of Corinthians, is a message to believing Christians!

These instructions about warring against the principalities and powers, casting down high things, and discerning spirits were not sent to people out in the world. They were sent to the saints. This fact should confirm that deliverance ministry belongs to the church and that freeing believers from the influence of demons is a vitally important act of service that edifies the body of Christ.

Here are a few more things to consider:
- The Great Commission found in Mark 16 says that those who believe in Jesus will cast out demons as a sign of their faith. Does this passage specify that Christians will only cast demons out of unbelievers? Or do we have to approach it with that presupposition in order to limit it that way?
- John 14:12 says that Christians will do the same work that Jesus did – a great deal of which involved freeing people from demons. Granted, Jesus only cast demons out of non-Christians because Christianity did not yet exist. Nevertheless, the model He gives us is that many times, people *with faith* need to be freed from demonic oppression (see Luke 8:40-48 and Luke 13:10-13 for just two examples).
- 1 Corinthians 6:19 describes the believer's body as a temple of the Holy Spirit. When Jesus drove the money changers from the physical temple, this could represent the believer's need to chase demons from our temple as well.

If I have demons, does that mean I am possessed?

No. It means you have given influence, power, and agreement over to the servants of Satan so that they have legal right to affect your life in negative ways. *Shadow Boxing* explains this quite well using the analogy of open doors. Sin, for example, is one way a believer can open a door for demons to come in. When we step out from God's protection through disobedience, that provides opportunity to the enemy.

The moment you were saved, you became the purchased possession of Jesus Christ (1 Corinthians 6:20). And yet, at the same time, believers who are honest with themselves can usually discern quite easily that certain areas of our lives are not in line with the will of our Lord. How can that be possible? How can the Holy Spirit inhabit the same person as a demon?

First, we must recognize that people are made in God's image. Part of the revelation God has released to His people is that just as He is Father, Son, and Holy Spirit all in one, we are spirit, soul, and body all in one (1 Thessalonians 5:23). The three main parts of the Old Testament temple represent a picture of this truth. The outer court represents the body. The Holy Place represents the soul, and the Holy of Holies represents the spirit.

The body consists of our physical makeup. Our flesh, bones, nerves, and systems make up the body. The soul consists of our mind, will, and emotions. Our spirit, or our innermost being, is the place of communion with God through the Holy Spirit. This is the part of humankind that died when Adam sinned, and that is born again when we receive Jesus as Lord.

With these things in mind, it is easy to see that our spirit is the place where Jesus has absolute dominion. The enemy cannot touch this holy place where the Lord's glory is. However, just as some ungodly men moved into the physical temple, sometimes the enemy can move into our body and soul. The body and soul are where demons can build their strongholds and affect a believer's life.

This brief explanation shows how someone can be born again and yet still suffer from demonic influence and oppression. It also explains how evil spirits can dwell in the same person as the Holy Spirit – they're not in the same part.

So again, the goal is to remove everything that is not of the Lord so that what is true in our spirits, the complete reign of Jesus Christ, becomes true in our souls and bodies as well. That is the true definition of freedom.

How can I be sure deliverance ministry will work?

Deliverance ministry is a powerful force in the lives of believers who trust in the working of Jesus. Jesus wants us free, so we can trust that He is working with us to make us completely free. Philippians 1:6 promises that the Lord will continue to perfect us until He comes again. So your first assurance that it will work is that Jesus wants it to work.

Moreover, when you allow Holy Spirit to search you and know you intimately, to show you what you have working against your destiny and calling, and when you respond, transformation will happen. Jesus said knowing the truth makes us free (John 8:32). Part of knowing the truth is allowing Him to show you exactly what things in your life are not of Him, and then receiving His power to be free.

Here are some reassurances:
- Matthew 28:18 says Jesus has all authority in Heaven and on Earth. There's none left for the devil except however much we give him by obeying him. The authority of Jesus means we can be free.
- Colossians 1:13-14 assures us that Jesus has rescued us from the rule of darkness.
- Romans 7:14 promises that sin shall no longer have dominion over us.
- Colossians 2:9-15 paints a picture of a completely victorious Jesus and an utterly humiliated enemy.
- Ephesians 1:3 says we are blessed with every spiritual blessing in the heavenly places. Surely that includes

freedom from demons.
- Ephesians 3:10 proclaims that the church gets to make Gods marvelous wisdom known to the principalities and powers. In other words, we get to show them who our God is, which is bad news for them.

The most important keys for successful deliverance are openness, honesty before God, humility, and faith. Being open allows God to search and root out all that is not of Him. Honesty means that when God does show us something, we do not deny it or justify it, but rather confess it, repent of it, receive forgiveness for it, and put it to death. Humility helps us acknowledge our need for the forgiveness, mercy, healing, and revival that only God can bring us. It also makes us more willing to *receive* these things. Finally, we must believe that God is doing what we are praying for (Matthew 21:20-22).

If you truly believe that God will do what He said He would do, you can rest assured that deliverance ministry will set you on new heights in your walk with the Lord.

Is deliverance a one-time thing?

I'm sure that it could be, but my experience and that of basically every solid Christian I know suggest that it is better to see deliverance as a lifestyle. We constantly allow Holy Spirit to show us things at work, and we are constantly delivered of those things the enemy intends for our harm.

One helpful concept is to view deliverance as peeling off layers. We peel back one layer of strongholds and demons, after which another layer becomes apparent. Layer by layer, the Lord takes us higher and deeper into the freedom He intends for us. Sometimes, we can rebuild things that we have previously destroyed. Sometimes, the enemy launches a new attack that we must battle through. There is no one-size-fits-all understanding of how deliverance may go or when it may become necessary.

We trust in this: Holy Spirit knows what He is doing. He knows what, when, where, and how to best set us free every single time. Why doesn't He just do it all at once? Honestly,

I do not know. But I am confident that there must be a good reason.

I've heard it said of the blessings of the Lord that if He were to pour out all the blessing He intended for us at one time, we'd explode. I don't know if that's true or not, but it very well could be. I believe deliverance is the same way: if God tried to tear down all that needed to be torn down and cast out everything that needed to be cast out all at once, it would likely be an overwhelming experience. I also believe that God allows us to walk the process out as a way to train us to listen, trust, and follow Him.

He's a good Dad, and He knows exactly what we need.

To the Wives and Family Members
Written by Karen McSpadden

I wish I didn't have to write this, and that you weren't having to read it. Believe me, I understand the heartbreak that comes from discovering your husband's porn habit. Nevertheless, we must keep in mind that we are in a war, and it's not against our husbands, our sons, or our fathers. Rather, we battle an enemy who wars against their souls and ours (Ephesians 6:12). As with every aspect of our spiritual journey, we must choose how we engage in this battle. Will we allow the enemy of our souls to destroy our marriages, or will we fight back with all our strength? I, for one, have given the enemy enough ground and am picking up my sword in the fight to take back every last bit he's stolen and make him tuck his tail and run along the way. I invite you to do the same.*

While I am doing my best to fight as led by the Holy Spirit, I must admit that I never imagined I would be in this particular battle. I grew up naïve. I didn't realize pornography was such a huge problem. I only had a vague notion that there were "adult magazines" and that was about it. Once I started growing in understanding of deliverance and things of the Spirit, however, I started to learn pornography was more widespread than I knew, but it still didn't affect me...or so I thought.

Even after Kevin and I were dating, and he'd confessed a slip with porn, I still didn't quite understand it for what it was. I forgave him and moved on without much thought or concern. That started to change after we were married. When he first confessed ongoing participation with pornography and masturbation again after we'd been married for a while,

---
*Once again, we acknowledge and understand there are also women who have struggled and battled lust, pornography, masturbation, etc., and that your struggle can be just as devastating to your relationships. I am just writing from my perspective as a wife, but what I'm saying can just as easily be applied to husbands or other family members responding to the sin of pornography in our loved ones.

it made me question whether I was truly "enough" for him. I began to feel rejected by him due to his choosing those things instead of or in addition to me. It was no longer a minor issue that I could ignore, but one that hurt me deeply.

Let me emphasize that my husband is absolutely wonderful. I cannot imagine a better, more thoughtful and servant-hearted man for the Lord to choose for me. So I know his participation with pornography did not happen because he didn't love me or desire me as his wife. I had laid hold of that truth as we worked through an earlier confession of his sin. I had chosen to trust completely in his love for me. That's partially why, prior to the most recent bout with pornography that he shared in the beginning of this book, I was flying high. I really believed he had the whole lust and pornography issue beat, and that we'd never again have to have one of those conversations.

Then it happened.

I was completely blindsided. I don't think I hardly said anything to him immediately after he confessed. At that point, I wasn't even quietly or respectfully trying to contain anger. I just had absolutely nothing to say.

The weeks and months after that conversation are kind of a blur to me. I remember generally having lots of conversations, some which found me being gentle and full of grace, honoring him as a man of God and expressing forgiveness and respect for him. But in others, I would lose my carefully constructed, keep-it-together facade and either cry or hurl my hurt and frustration at him. To his credit, he never once fought back. He knew that even if my words weren't in the right spirit, he was the one who'd messed up, and he was walking out his own healing and restoration as he's shared so beautifully in this book. There was probably a three to four month period that was the most challenging time we've walked through in 8 years of marriage. But it was in that time that I learned to walk in my own freedom. I heard Jesus inviting me, "Buy from Me gold refined in the fire" (Revelation 3:18). Through His teaching, healing, and refining, I could finally allow myself to truly forgive my husband, be healed myself, and see our marriage restored and soaring.

THE FOUNDATION

I can truly testify of the goodness of God, that no matter how deep the betrayal, how repetitive the sin, how much of a mess you feel your marriage is in, that there's nothing Jesus cannot heal, forgive, and restore.

In John 10:10, Jesus says, "I have come that [you] may have life, and that [you] may have it more abundantly." Friends, Jesus understands betrayal. Just look at Judas Iscariot, one of the Lord's closest friends who sold Him out. Jesus understands believers' falling back into the same sins. Look at Peter and how many times in the Gospels his mouth got him in trouble. Furthermore, Jesus understands a marriage where one partner isn't living up to his or her part of the covenant. Look at the body of Christ, His Bride. Some of us may be great wives to Jesus, but others who claim to belong to Him look to Him alone to sustain the relationship instead of continually nurturing it together.

An important first step is to come out of agreement with the lie that Jesus can't understand how we are feeling about what our spouse or loved one has done. He knows how we feel, and He is able to help us overcome our situation. That is, He can help us if we let Him. Instead of wallowing in the muck of hurt feelings and frustrations, let's agree with Him and His Word that He "is able to do exceedingly abundantly above all that we ask or think, according to [His] power that works in us" (Ephesians 3:20). After all, His power alone can restore our marriages not only to what they were, but to what God Himself dreams and desires for them to be.

I don't know about you, but I want a dynamite marriage, period. That requires a partnership, and the very word partnership implies by definition at least two people. The covenant partnership of marriage guarantees that just as both of you will enjoy each other's triumphs together, you will also endure each other's failures and bad choices together.

Now, your husband's fall into these areas of sexual immorality is not your fault. I need you to have that established first. Never hear me say in any way that his choices are your fault. But, once he has confessed and shown true repentance (a change in heart and behavior, turning and going the other direction), then if you choose to hold onto the unforgiveness, bitterness, hurt, anger, and betrayal you feel in your heart, my friend, you are now part of the problem instead of the solution!

Jesus tells a parable in Matthew 18:21-35 about a servant who has his large debt forgiven, but then does not return the favor to a fellow servant who owed a small amount. In this parable, He says that the one who did not forgive the debt was "delivered... to the torturers," and "so My heavenly Father also will do to you if each of you, from his heart, does not forgive his brother his trespasses" (verses 34-35). Had I not chosen forgiveness every single time the enemy wanted to come at me with accusations about my husband, well, I just don't want to think about the possibilities. Continuing to participate with unforgiveness toward my husband in this one area, even though I've been forgiven much, would have opened me up to torment from the enemy. I would have stepped outside the will of my Father who commands that we continue to forgive (Matthew 18:22), so He can also continue to forgive us (Matthew 6:14-15).

You might ask, "But isn't this sin of lust/pornography/masturbation/sexual immorality worse than anything I've ever done to him?" Dear friend, remember I'm not sharing anything I haven't had to learn myself, and that mindset is nothing but grade-A pride, which is also sin. The book of 1 John 1:8 says "If we say that we have no sin, we deceive ourselves, and the truth is not in us." Romans 3:23 reminds us that "all have sinned and fall short of the glory of God," and Romans 6:23 makes clear that "the wages of sin is death." Sometimes in our woundedness, we want to justify staying angry at our husbands for their sin against God and us, because when we are angry, we can hide from the hurt we feel. But I don't get to judge my husband for what he's done. That is actually the worst type of pride, to put myself in God's place of judgment.

In this light, holding on to pride and unforgiveness is no better or worse than your husband's participation with pornography. In fact, in Mark 7:20-23, as Jesus lists things within the heart that defile us, He includes pride right after adultery and fornication. Proverbs 6:16-19 lists a proud look as the first of an inventory of things that God hates and sees as an abomination. Psalm 101:5 clearly states, "The one who has a haughty look and a proud heart, him I will not endure." There are dozens more Scriptures that detail the snare that is pride. For our purposes, these verses are enough evidence to show us that it is essential to recognize pride in operation. We have to choose to repent from our own pride to begin to see healing and restoration in our hearts and relationships. "For if we sin willfully after we have received the knowledge of the truth, there no longer remains a sacrifice for sins" (Hebrews 10:26).

These truths lead us to the following exhortation: "Therefore humble yourselves under the mighty hand of God, that He may exalt you in due time, casting all your care upon Him, for He cares for you" (1 Peter 5:6-7). Your journey to healing in your own heart and in your marriage starts with recognizing and repenting for your own pride, so that you can then choose to forgive your husband. We have to always remember forgiveness doesn't mean what the other person did was okay, but it allows you to release your own hurt, anger, etc., and allow Jesus to take it.

Practically speaking, as you go through your day, if an accusation comes at you, just speak out (or whisper under your breath, or go to the restroom or your car if you are at work), "I choose to forgive (name) for stumbling into pornography. It made me feel (insert your true feelings here, and be specific. For example, "betrayed" or "not desired"). Jesus, I choose to receive Your healing and wholeness." Don't merely ask God to help you forgive him; it's your choice to forgive him and release him, and to give your hurt to the Lord. Remember, your choice to forgive is also your choice to partner with God and your spouse's repentant heart to restore your marriage.

You may need to repeatedly remind yourself that your husband is forgiven as you walk through healing and allow the Holy Spirit to uncover the depths at which your soul (your mind, will, and emotions) has been wounded. Remember that this is a battle, and don't be discouraged as you continue to fight. The enemy of your soul hates seeing you healed and delivered from torment, so he will likely try to bring accusations to you about your husband. After all, he is the accuser of the brethren (Rev 12:10). Therefore, as you overcome, it's important to literally speak out the truth, such as "My husband is forgiven, in Jesus name. Those sins are under the blood of Jesus." Just as Kevin wrote about how speaking out things coming against him destroyed their power, to speak out that you have forgiven your husband will destroy the lies and schemes of the enemy that want to keep you bound in your pain and brokenness. There is greater and deeper healing that the Father wants to accomplish to make you whole again, and it starts with standing on the foundation of forgiveness.

WALK IT OUT

Philippians 2:12-13 says that we work out our own salvation, as God is also working in us. If you read Appendix 1 of this book, it explains to us that salvation also means we are healed and made whole in every way, not just that we will go to Heaven when we die. So to say that we are walking out our salvation in this journey of healing in our relationships is certainly accurate.

Have you ever gone on a walk? Perhaps around your neighborhood for a little exercise, or a long walk on the beach or in the woods, or maybe just extra walking around your local mall trying to find the perfect gift for a loved one?

Regardless of the distance, any walk requires two consistent things - taking one step at a time, and continuing to put one foot in front of the other. This journey, too, requires us to take one step at a time, and to keep on going. I want to share with you some practical things I learned in my own personal journey of walking out healing and restoration.

Talk often, and be honest about your struggles and challenges as you walk things out from your side of his sin. However, be respectful towards your husband and don't pile on him. Do speak out what you know is true about him, or even what you want to be true of him. For example, you can affirm that he is a good and godly man, that he is honorable, that he is pure, that he is devoted to you and your family, etc. He needs to feel safe and encouraged, just like you do. Don't use his sin as a weapon weeks, months, or years later during a disagreement or fight. It's not fair to him, and let's be honest – we wouldn't like it if the tables were turned and he brought up our past sins and mistakes. Remember, this one sin is not the be-all, end-all sin unless you choose to give it that kind of power over your marriage.

Get with a trusted person in your life, such as a pastor or spiritual mentor, to help pray with you and counsel you personally. You need to have someone who will love you and encourage you, allow you to cry and vent, but also be willing to shoot you straight when it's needed. You need someone you can trust if they bring correction or call you out on unforgiveness, bitterness, etc. Some couples may also want or need to work on some marriage issues together in a counseling type setting. Once again, I would recommend a pastor or spiritual mentor versus just a "marriage counselor," because we know and understand that there are spiritual roots at work to cause these problems for your husband. Moreover, if you have marriage relationship issues aside from his sexual sin, then there are going to be similar roots behind those issues, too, that someone with discernment can help you uproot together.

Ask your husband how you can help him and pray for him. It disarms the enemy's attacks against you when you go before the King on your husband's behalf. It also makes it a lot easier to have grace towards him when you are praying for him. It is much more difficult to stay mad at your husband while genuinely praying for him. I'm not talking about the prayers that come from hurt and frustration, such as, "God show him where he was wrong and how he needs to make it up." I'm talking about prayer that earnestly seeks God's best for your husband. If he comes to you and asks you to pray for him, pray out loud right then and there; it will strengthen him to overcome, and empower you both to trample on the works and schemes of the enemy.

Never jump on him or fuss at him if he does share that he is feeling tempted or asks specifically for prayer. You have to choose to trust, just like you have to choose to forgive. It takes time to build trust again, but to build it you have to choose to start somewhere, and choose to keep building just like you choose to keep walking.

Talk together about practical things to help him avoid temptation and help you feel secure. For example, Kevin mentioned that he has asked me to disable the internet browser on his phone if I'm traveling for work without him. He has also chosen on his own to delete apps off his phone where he cannot control content others post or ads that may pop up with questionable images. For you, or your husband, that may look differently; talk together to figure out what he feels will help cut the tips off those hooks that want to catch him. Respect whatever he feels is important, and don't feel suspicious towards him based on his choices. For example, if he says he doesn't want to go to the community pool this summer, don't assume that means he has always checked out other women there before. He may just want to remove those opportunities for temptation for a season.

Don't share his issues, your hurt feelings, and your marriage issues with your mother, your girlfriends, your co-workers, etc. Women tend to process our feelings by talking through them, but that doesn't mean we need to drag our heart issues through the mud with anyone who will listen. Your mom and your girlfriends may be trusted and they may mean well, but they'll also be the ones who will be upset with your husband on your behalf, and they won't always hear how things are turning around for good. Let's be honest, sometimes this is a flaw for us as women; we want to vent the negative but we don't always come back and share the positive. Some of the best pre-marriage advice I received was from a spiritual mom who told me, "I don't want to know about Kevin hurting your feelings and you guys having a fight, because then you'll have already made up, and I'll still be mad at him on your behalf." This is why I encourage you instead to share your heart with a trusted mentor or pastor whom you can count on to be objective and seek Holy Spirit. These mentors are more likely to provide you with godly counsel than a close friend or family member who wants to try to make you feel better. Even if friends or family members are also mature believers, it's just always harder to be objective when someone we are close to is sharing a hurt caused by someone else.

Don't avoid or ignore him, physically or emotionally. There may be times when you want to be nowhere near him, or you don't want him to touch you, even to hold your hand or put an arm around you, much less any kind of deeper intimacy. But don't make this a habit that you fall into regularly. Your marriage cannot heal if you choose to isolate yourself from your husband. It's also against the Word; did you know the Bible actually teaches married couples to remain physically intimate? First Corinthians 7:3-5 teaches that in a marriage, husbands and wives should take care of one another's needs, that we each have authority over the others' bodies, and that we ought not deprive one another unless for a short time to focus on prayer and fasting. Even then we're exhorted to come back together so Satan does not tempt us. I would recommend reading this passage in the New Living Translation of the Bible – it puts it very plainly in our modern everyday language.

THE VICTORIOUS LIFE

Kevin has shared how deception works on the men to ensnare them. But friends, the enemy is not nearly as creative he'd like us to believe. He uses similar schemes on the women. Put yourself in a similar mindset to what Kevin laid out for men on page 25, but let's look at a woman's thought process when we let that runaway train derail in our minds.

You may find yourself thinking: He has let me down and hurt me before. It's only a matter of time before he does it again. What is he looking at so intently over there on his phone, anyways? Or perhaps for you it may sound more like this: Am I not enough for him? Am I not beautiful enough, thin enough, desirable enough? Does he even still want me sexually? Does he even love me? Did he ever really love me, or is that why he did this to me? I bet some of that sounds familiar.

Just as Kevin described for the guys, when we choose to pay attention to those things instead of shutting them down and refusing to give our attention to it, it hooks us. We are tempted into sin, such as bitterness, unforgiveness, isolation, participating with ungodly grief, depression, and more when we give our attention to these thoughts and allow them to continue to marinate in our minds. If we are honest with ourselves, allowing these ungodly thoughts to continue circulating is just a different twist on a fantasy, which is simply defined as an idea with no basis in reality (dictionary.com).

As Kevin explained in this book, deception works to trick, scare, or threaten you into keeping your struggles to yourself. That's why honest communication with your husband is so important. I didn't have to give him all the gory details of my mental runaway mind train, but I did have to tell him that I was struggling with thoughts coming against me, or to accuse him, in order to expose them for the lies they were and give him opportunity to speak truth. We overcome Satan by the blood of the Lamb, Jesus Christ, and by the words of

His, and of our, testimony (Revelation 12:11)!

I want you to imagine that someone insulted your husband and attacked his character right in front of you. How would you respond to that individual? I would hope you'd quickly correct them, stand up for your man, and tell them just how great he is and how wrong they are about their judgments toward him. So ladies, when the enemy wants to attack your husband and bring accusations against him in your mind, don't agree with those lies, but give that dumb devil what for! You tell him who God made your husband to be, and how great God is at bringing healing and restoration, and that he may have come at you that one way, but he will soon tuck his tail and run and flee any way he can (Deuteronomy 28:7).

Part two of this book also describes endurance and vigilance, and how these things are important to continue overcoming areas that had led to bondage, sin, and death in the past. Friends, it is just as important for us as wives to maintain steadfast endurance and vigilance in our own hearts and minds against the schemes of the devil to shatter our marriages. Remember the lesson on the bombardment? Satan is methodical in his schemes against us. He looks for a weak spot in our wall against his attacks, and then he will hit it over and over again unless we deal with the weak spot.

Do you have any unforgiveness anywhere? Have you participated with one of those runaway mind train accusations? Are you partnering with doubt against your husband's faithfulness without cause? You have to be willing to open your heart to the Holy Spirit to search you and know you, and then allow Him to uproot anything that is not of Him (Psalm 139:23-24). You have to choose to do what I just described above and literally speak out truth so that you can overcome. You have to repent for where you've participated and agreed with doubt, ungodly sorrow, or whatever it is.

Kevin gave examples for guys where vigilance is vital for them to avoid falling back into temptation and sin (page 66). I could make a case that the same principles are true for us as women. We must remain vigilant in order to avoid falling back under the devil's bombardment and actively participating with those same old self-destructive, marriage-killing thought patterns and arguments. As Kevin said, emotionally intense situations can put us in a state where we become vulnerable to the enemy's attacks. We must always remember to listen to the voice of Holy Spirit, as He will guide us into all truth (John 16:13). When you hear that Voice, you must choose to listen and to obey what He is telling you to do. Endurance and vigilance both really come down to focusing our gaze on Jesus, instead of the circumstances of the moment, the emotional state of our hearts, or the barrage of negative thoughts bombarding our minds.

Finally, as wives we too must stand fast. We too should pay attention to the warning of Paul in 1 Corinthians 10:12: "Therefore, let him who thinks he stands, take heed lest he fall." Just as our husbands cannot become complacent in their hearts and minds in overcoming lust and temptation to sexual sin, we as their wives cannot become complacent in praying for them and for our marriages. We must stand steadfast in our own hearts and minds against the devil's accusations and schemes. It is a beautiful and powerful thing to be his helper. We were created for this, from the very beginning. In Genesis 2:18 God decided it was not good for Adam to be alone, and created woman (Eve), to be his helpmate, the meaning of which includes being his friend, companion, and helper. Let us not lay down the roles we were created for, but let us run with them, pouring all of our passion into them, and loving and trusting Father God every step of the way. Watch how He will heal and bless your marriage as you continue to love, honor, serve, pray for, encourage, and gird up your husband. Watch how He takes your struggles and trials the two of you had to walk through and turns ashes into beauty. And watch Him prove His Word in your lives: "Behold, I am the Lord, the God of all flesh. Is there anything too hard for Me?" (Jeremiah 32:27)

Great grace to you, my friend, and may the God of peace be with you. May He bless you, keep you, and make His face to shine upon you.

Karen McSpadden

WEAPONS OF OUR WARFARE:

Humbling ourselves means we obey what God's written and revealed word say to do. Pride says "I want," while humility says, "yes, Lord."

WEAPONS OF OUR WARFARE:

God has given us tools and weapons that work to destroy the enemy's power. It is up to use to USE those weapons by the direction of the Holy Spirit.

LIBERATED

WEAPONS OF OUR WARFARE:

Choice. *Our choices determine what power operates in our lives. Choosing to obey God makes us free from sin's power and helps us grow in His. Submitting to sin increases its power over us. The constant choice to obey God is a mighty weapon in our arsenal.*

WEAPONS OF OUR WARFARE:

Secrecy is never the right choice when it comes to temptation or sin. Secrecy tends to lead to isolation. Divide and conquer is one of the oldest – and most effective – plays in the enemy's book.

WEAPONS OF OUR WARFARE:

Obedience. *Ever notice how often obedience or the lack thereof makes all the difference? That's why Jesus gave us the model: I speak what I hear my Father speaking; I do what I see Him doing. If it worked for Jesus...*

WEAPONS OF OUR WARFARE:

Know your weaknesses and act accordingly. If you're aware of how you might be tempted, you have the power to remove that option from the table. Enough said.

LIBERATED

WEAPONS OF OUR WARFARE:

Allowing the Holy Spirit to reveal our rightful place in the body of Christ and to show us how God sees us accomplishes two things: 1. It destroys the notion that we're not important to Him. 2. It forces us to humble ourselves as we depend on Him to transform us into the ones He created us to be.

WEAPONS OF OUR WARFARE:

Confessing sin, repenting (committing to yourself and to Jesus that you fully intend to turn away from sin and toward His purposes and plans), and receiving the discipline of the Lord are powerful weapons in your arsenal. While many do not think of these vital acts as warfare, each of them plays a role in restoring your right relationship, both with God and man. Furthermore, they each help you solidify your true identity in Him, which increases your power to overcome the temptation to sin in the future.

WEAPONS OF OUR WARFARE:

John 14:12 says, "most assuredly, I say to you, he who believes in Me, the works that I do he will do also; and greater works than these he will do, because I go to My Father." This is Jesus's personal guarantee that He empowers us to walk in His freedom.

WEAPONS OF OUR WARFARE:

Prayer of Faith. The prayers in this section will have as much power as you have faith in what the Lord will do. It is pointless to simply say words. Put your trust in what Jesus said, that if we ask and do not doubt, it will be done for us.

WEAPONS OF OUR WARFARE:

Choices. Since Satan cannot force saints to act according to his will, we always get to choose. God provides the way out. When we choose to follow God's way, deliberately and with determination, we effectively resist the devil. It is dangerous to postpone the choice. A friend of mine is fond of telling her kids, "Obey, right away, without delay." That saying applies in these situations as well.

WEAPONS OF OUR WARFARE:

Which conversation are you having? Jesus stayed in communion with the Father at all times, and even in temptation, only spoke to the enemy to release the Word of God. Arguing with the enemy is a trap. It is far more powerful to remain in constant conversation with your loving Father and only speak to the enemy as you release what God says toward him. When temptation comes, simply speak to the Lord instead. Try something along these lines: "Father I affirm You as Lord of my life, eternal, and all powerful. Thank You for the revenge You will take on my enemies on my behalf. Your Word says I'm clean because You have spoken to me, and I proclaim my cleanness in Your sight due to the blood of Jesus. Thank You for cleansing and protecting me."

WEAPONS OF OUR WARFARE:

Meditate on what is good. Scripture commands followers of Jesus to meditate on what is good, noble, and lovely. This is analogous to filling a container – if my bucket is full of gold, there is no room for someone to put dirt in it. Similarly, if I fill my mind and heart with God's glory and the things of His kingdom, there's no room for the enemy's filth.

WEAPONS OF OUR WARFARE:

The Fear of the Lord. The fear of the Lord is a deep reverence for Who He is. It is an intense honor for the character and the ways of the Lord. Revering King Jesus, the Rider on the white horse from whose mouth the two-edged sword proceeds, will never lead you wrong. Ask the Holy Spirit on a regular basis to release to you a fresh impartation of the fear of the Lord.

LIBERATED

WEAPONS OF OUR WARFARE:

How do you attack while staying protected? One of the best ways is to release God's angels to carry out His Word against the enemy. Psalm 103:20 says they obey the voice of His Word. These mighty and vicious warriors are more than willing to go destroy the emissaries of the enemy before they ever have a chance to get to you. So practically speaking, follow these steps. 1. Speak out and agree with God's Word as led by the Holy Spirit. 2. Dispatch the angels assigned to you to go and carry out God's Word according to His will, in the name of Jesus. 3. Thank God for His mighty hosts who perform His Word.

📖 STRONGHOLD:

a place where the believer has surrendered authority to the enemy; a pattern of thoughts, behaviors, or words that has power and gains more power the longer a believer allows it to exist. Think of it as a place where demonic spirits can "live," or occupy space in your life.

📖 RENOUNCE:

According to Dictionary.com, to renounce something means:

1. *to give up or put aside voluntarily.*
2. *to give up by formal declaration.*
3. *to repudiate; disown. In other words, you renounce something when you willfully decide to put it away and give up ownership or participation with it.*

LIBERATED

DEVASTATING CYCLE

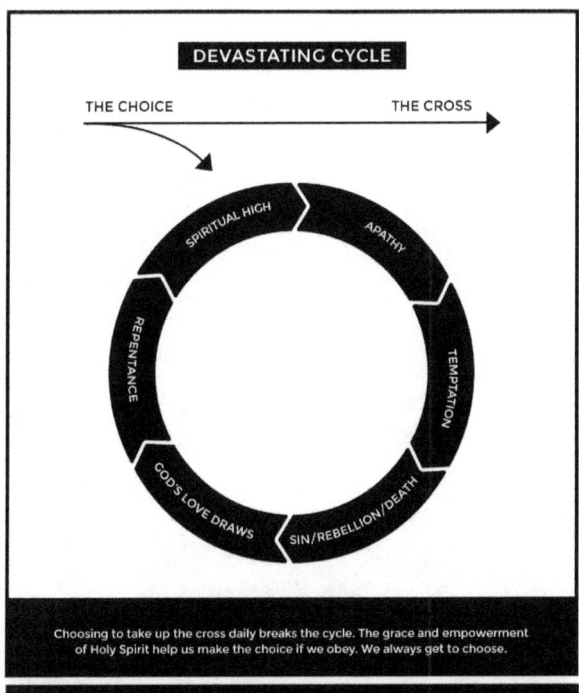

THE CHOICE → THE CROSS

- SPIRITUAL HIGH
- APATHY
- TEMPTATION
- SIN/REBELLION/DEATH
- GOD'S LOVE DRAWS
- REPENTANCE

Choosing to take up the cross daily breaks the cycle. The grace and empowerment of Holy Spirit help us make the choice if we obey. We always get to choose.

DECEPTION AND THE JAMES 1 PROCESS

Deception is a slippery slope. The further you go, the harder it is to climb out.

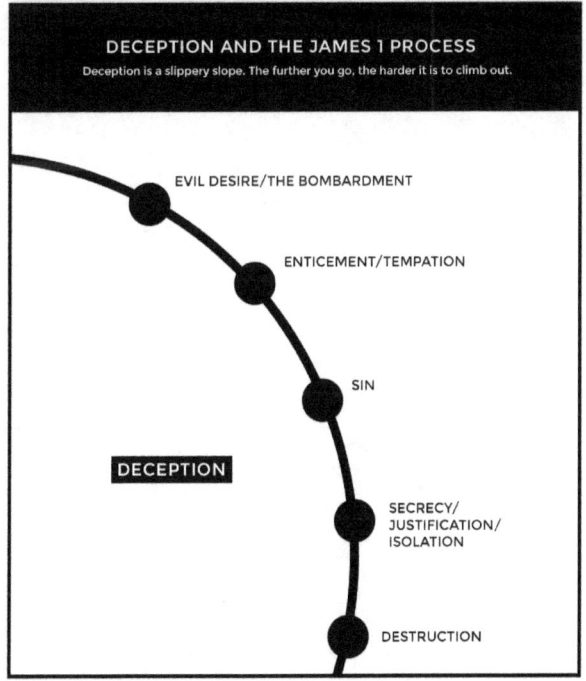

- EVIL DESIRE/THE BOMBARDMENT
- ENTICEMENT/TEMPTATION
- SIN

DECEPTION

- SECRECY/JUSTIFICATION/ISOLATION
- DESTRUCTION

LIBERATED

1

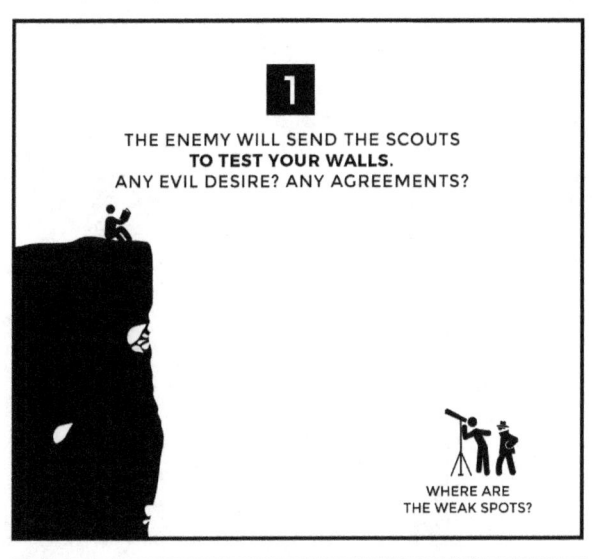

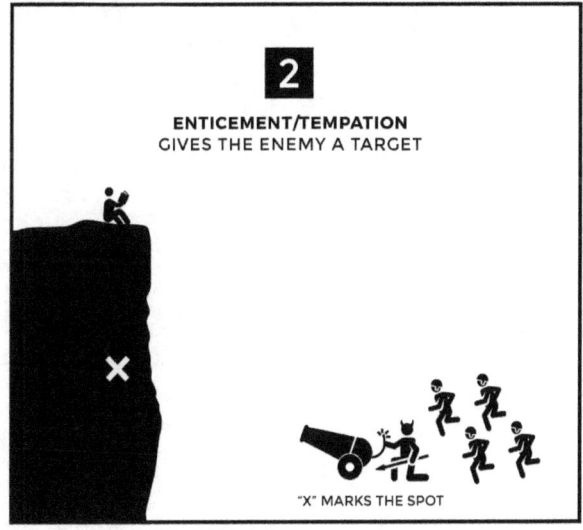

THE ENEMY WILL SEND THE SCOUTS TO TEST YOUR WALLS.
ANY EVIL DESIRE? ANY AGREEMENTS?

WHERE ARE THE WEAK SPOTS?

2

ENTICEMENT/TEMPATION
GIVES THE ENEMY A TARGET

"X" MARKS THE SPOT

LIBERATED

3
THE BOMBARDMENT BEGINS
AND **THE BATTLE IS ON**

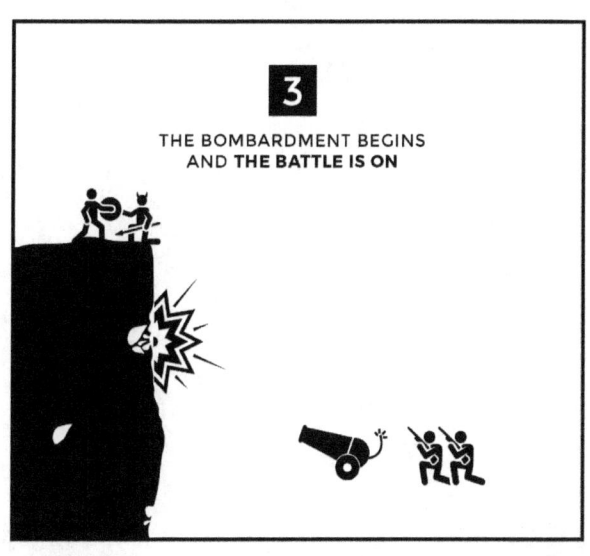

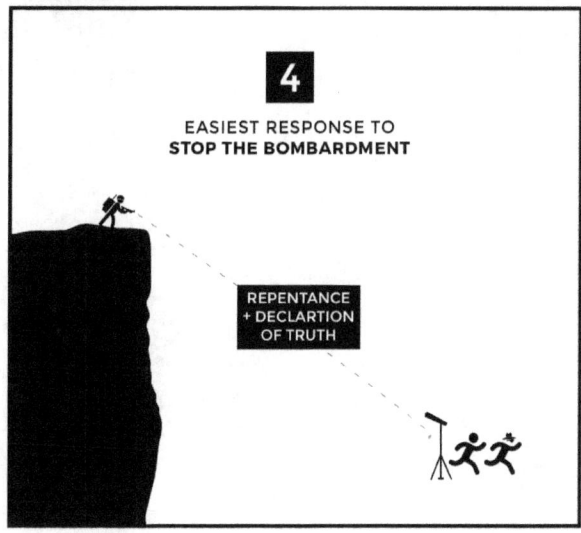

4
EASIEST RESPONSE TO
STOP THE BOMBARDMENT

REPENTANCE
+ DECLARTION
OF TRUTH

LIBERATED

THE BEST DEFENSE

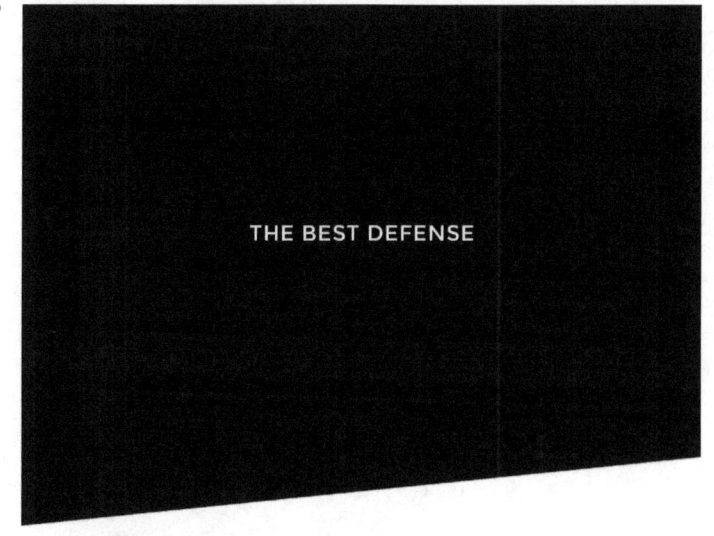

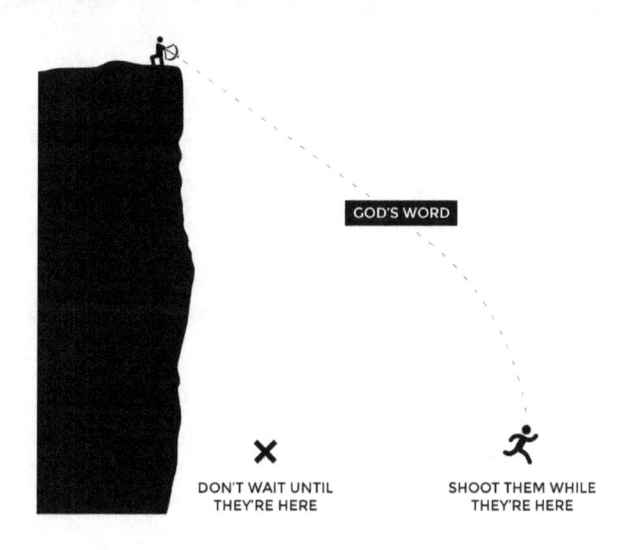

GOD'S WORD

✗ DON'T WAIT UNTIL THEY'RE HERE

🏃 SHOOT THEM WHILE THEY'RE HERE

LIBERATED

KINGDOM OF HEAVEN

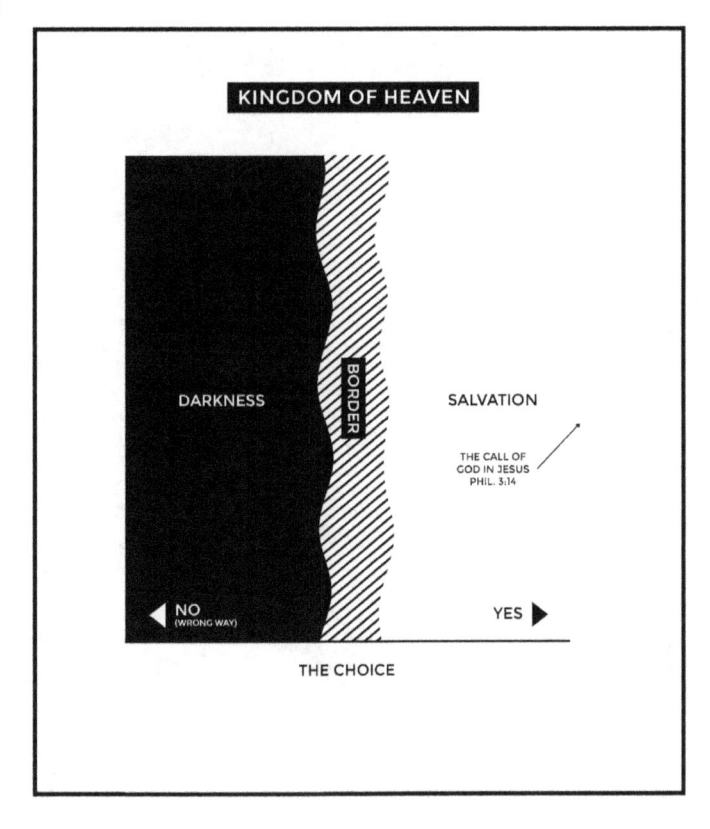

DARKNESS

BORDER

SALVATION

THE CALL OF
GOD IN JESUS
PHIL. 3:14

◀ **NO**
(WRONG WAY)

YES ▶

THE CHOICE

LIBERATED

ABOUT THE AUTHOR

Karen and Kevin McSpadden serve on the leadership team at the Garden Gathering Church in San Angelo, Texas. They are committed to helping others discover the freedom and healing they have received from the Lord Jesus by the power of the Holy Spirit.

LIBERATED

GARDENPUBLISHINGCO.COM

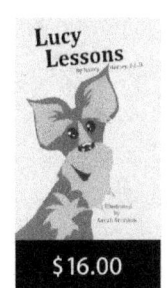

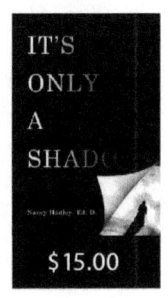

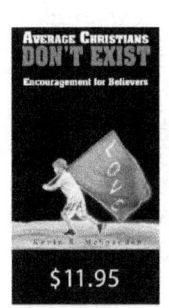

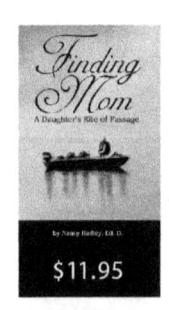

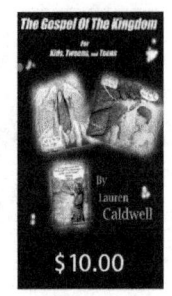

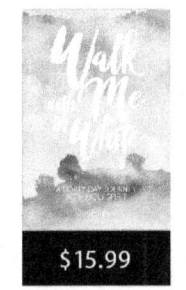

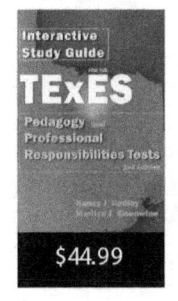

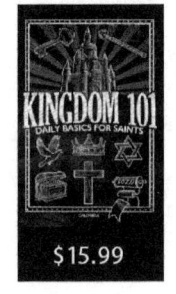

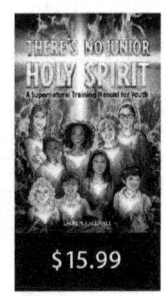

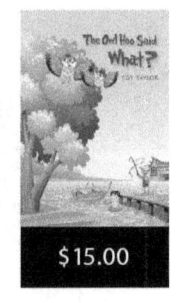

Lucy Lessons — $16.00	IT'S ONLY A SHADOW — $15.00	Finding Mom: A Daughter's Rite of Passage — $11.95
Average Christians Don't Exist: Encouragement for Believers — $11.95	The Gospel Of The Kingdom for Kids, Tweens, and Teens by Lauren Caldwell — $10.00	Walk With Me — $15.99
Kingdom 101: Daily Basics for Saints — $15.99	Interactive Study Guide TExES Pedagogy and Professional Responsibilities Tests — $44.99	There's No Junior Holy Spirit: A Supernatural Training Manual for Youth — $15.99
The Owl Hoo Said What? — $15.00		

CPSIA information can be obtained
at www.ICGtesting.com
Printed in the USA
LVHW012226180520
655844LV00006B/745

9 780996 645348